Advance Praise

"Prostate cancer and its treatments can have significant effects on a man's sexuality, but there's not much information about that for anyone, much less gay men. Gerald Perlman has done an excellent job of bringing together physicians, therapists, researchers, and cancer survivors, giving gay a complete picture of the issues and concerns they may face. Through frank discussion and personal accounts, each chapter offers different perspectives on the options men have and the choices they make. The medical section gives a remarkably complete picture of treatment possibilities, the current research and understanding of prostate cancer, and how it affects gay men. In the experiential section, prostate cancer survivors share their stories, how they made treatment decisions, and how it affected their relationships. They also give plenty of tips for navigating the healthcare system, minimizing post-surgery discomfort, talking with sexual partners, and more. Almost one out of three gay couples will experience prostate cancer. What Every Gay Man Needs to Know about Prostate Cancer has the information you need to deal with it."

—Charlie Glickman, PhD and Aislinn Emirzian, authors of *The Ultimate Guide to Prostate Pleasure*

WHAT EVERY GAY MAN NEEDS TO KNOW ABOUT PROSTATE CANCER

GERALD PERLMAN, PHD

This book is not a substitute for professional medical advice from a healthcare professional. All concerns regarding one's physical well-being, including diagnosis and treatment of any condition in need of medical attention, should be directed to a trained physician and/or healthcare provider. The goal of this book is only to help individuals make the choices that are perhaps best for them under the care of a healthcare professional.

Magnus Books , An Imprint of Riverdale Avenue Books
5676 Riverdale Avenue, Suite 101
New York, NY 10471
www.riverdaleavebooks.com

First Edition
ISBN: 978-1-936833-05-4

Dedicated to

Bert Schaffner, MD
(1913-2010)

Mentor, colleague, friend, inspiration

Table of Contents

Part Two
*Experiential Section: Gay Men Write about Their Own
Experiences of Coping with Prostate Cancer*

Introduction

Why a Book about Prostate Cancer for Gay Men?

Gerald Perlman, PhD

After I was diagnosed with prostate cancer (PCa) in August 2000, I experienced what could be called an acute stress disorder followed by several months of which, in retrospect, might be described as a post-traumatic stress disorder (PSTD). In my distress, I searched for a self-help group in New York City (where I live and work) that catered to gay men who have been diagnosed with and/or treated for PCa. At the time, only one such group existed in the entire country; that was Malecare. In addition to providing a monthly lecture series, Darryl Mitteldorf, a straight man who founded Malecare to serve all men struggling with a variety of cancers, led a weekly group for men diagnosed with PCa and a monthly supplementary group specifically for gay men.

I have chronicled the journey of going from group member to group facilitator in an essay in a book entitled *A Gay Man's Guide to Prostate Cancer*. Since the book's publication in 2005, I have received inquiries, praise, and sometimes hate mail asking why such a book was necessary. "After all," the question goes, "isn't biology biology whether gay or straight?" And the answer is: Of course, but during and following the initial prostate cancer diagnosis and after treatment, many similarities between the experiences of gay and straight men diverge.

Until diagnosed, prostate cancer is off most people's radar screens. When the newly diagnosed seek treatment information from professional publications and the Internet, they will find information almost entirely written by, for, and about heterosexual men and their female partners. Gay and bisexual men find almost nothing written by, for, or about them.

As suggested in a recent article in the *New York Times*, most urologists assume their patients are heterosexual and are either ignorant of or uncomfortable with gay men's issues in general, and about their particular concerns regarding prostate cancer. The typical gay, bisexual, or transgender (male-to-female) patient fills out registration forms and inventories that include no questions about sexual orientation or identity, sees no literature in the waiting-room written for gay people, and ends his first meeting with the urologist without ever having been asked about his sexual orientation or identity. Gay men typically have to adapt to largely heterosexual settings in most areas of health care services. The gay patient typically leaves the consultation room with his unique questions unanswered: Which treatment will allow me to continue to experience receptive and/or insertive anal intercourse? Which treatment might preserve my ejaculate, and if I choose a treatment that leaves me with no cum, how might my sex partner(s) and I react? What if my penis never again gets hard enough to penetrate a man's anus, which is quite different from having the ability to penetrate a vagina? What are the effects of anal intercourse on prostate-specific antigen (PSA) readings? Is there a correlation between anal intercourse and PCa? How long must one wait after treatment to engage in anal stimulation of any sort? How will the absence of a prostate gland affect anal pleasure? What are the complications if one has HIV/AIDS in addition to prostate cancer? Will my sperm be saved in case I want to have kids? Will I even be asked about saving my sperm? Will the size of my penis shrink after surgery? And the list goes on for each individual gay man. The undercurrent of ignorance that gay men might innocently, or not so innocently, face during their urological consultations is often upsetting, dehumanizing, and even enraging. It is often experienced as marginalizing, dismissive and/or humiliating. Many gay men, as an already marginalized and stigmatized group, are afraid to speak up about their concerns. The situation puts the onus on the patient to ask the questions that they may be too frightened and/or ashamed to ask.

Socially, gay men live in a world burnished by over thirty years of HIV/AIDS: illness, activism and death. As gay men navigate the heterosexually-biased world of prostate cancer treatment, they must simultaneously confront potential problems of stigmatization within the context of the gay community itself regarding post-treatment scarring, ejaculation deficits, erectile dysfunction, incontinence, coming out again (this time as someone who has prostate cancer), and/or competing for attention and compassion living with HIV/AIDS.

It is well understood that most gay men harbor their own internalized homophobia and shame about their sexual orientation and desires. Gay men with prostate cancer often have to cope with shameful feelings, and feelings of inadequacy and undesirability resulting from the effects of treatment that may parallel the feelings that often accompany the formation of a gay identity. Much of that shame is expressed through concerns about the body: obsessions with flaws, the need to appear hyper-masculine, rejection of the effeminate and the over-weight, and the fear of aging, among others. Most gay men go through a process of feeling flawed or like "damaged goods." It is common knowledge that coping with HIV/ AIDS re-ignites and exacerbates these feelings. So, it seems clear that having to deal with the possible side effects of PCa treatment adds yet another layer of potentially shame-triggering issues with which the gay man has to deal.

3

In 2011, the American Cancer Society estimated that 217,000 American men would be diagnosed with prostate cancer. A 2011 newsletter from the Prostate Cancer Foundation highlighted the following key facts: Within the next 15.6 minutes, a man will die from prostate cancer; in the next 2.2 minutes, a man will be informed that he has prostate cancer; in America, men are 35% more likely to be diagnosed with prostate cancer than women are to develop breast cancer; more than 33,000 men will die from the disease; and the average American man has about a 16% chance of being diagnosed with prostate cancer during his lifetime. And although the rate of gay men diagnosed with or dying from PCa, as compared to their heterosexual counterparts, has not been studied, the impact on two men partnered and/or living together increases the odds of the effect PCa may have on gay men.

Gay and bisexual men diagnosed with prostate cancer face even more obstacles if they are from non-white minority groups. The risk of prostate cancer and mortality among African-Americans, for example, is significantly higher than it is for their white counterparts. African-American church congregations and community clinics have recently begun promoting public awareness about prostate cancer through special events and outreach programs. But gay men of color rarely find such community organizations welcoming or tolerant of them, and they are often shut out of these opportunities.

Whether living alone without a partner or living with one in a relationship, gay men face the same morbidity concerns that straight men do, though rarely with the same level of external support regarding their unique needs. It is not easy to find a place where gay men can talk about not being able to share ejaculate or an erect penis with a male sex-partner. Gay men diagnosed with prostate cancer also revisit the coming out experience they may have gone through years before. For various reasons related to coming out and best known to them, several men writing in the experiential section of this book have chosen to use pseudonyms, which are indicated by putting the author's name in quotation marks. Coming out as gay is difficult and may not be resolved for some of these men. Coming out about prostate cancer often re-traumatizes gay men. Every gay man goes through a process of first coming out to himself. Then he may come out to his family, friends, and colleagues, always with the dread of possible rejection, stigmatization, scorn and loss. The process can be painful, humiliating, and anger provoking. Coming out as a prostate cancer patient with its sexual overtones re-ignites that very experience and can often end with the same painful and shameful consequences. Straight men, in telling their loved ones, their friends, and/or their sex partners about their prostate cancer, typically have no comparable historical/psychological experience.

It is well documented that marginalized and stigmatized groups do better and feel freer expressing their fears and concerns, in addition to healing better, when in the presence of others like themselves. Peer support groups promote authentic identification with people like oneself (role models) and a safe and open environment in which to reveal one's particular fears and concerns. In a predominantly straight support group, issues of concern to gay men either do not get discussed or are given short shrift. Sometimes the experience is felt as harmful by the gay man who attempts to raise those issues that are worrisome to him. Thus, having a resource available to gay men is an invaluable tool to have as they struggle with the many choices and uncertainties that confront them once diagnosed with prostate cancer, or even before as they contemplate making a screening-appointment with a urologist. To be able to read material that is geared specifically toward gay men and written by gay men who have gone through the experience is an invaluable resource.

At the same time, much of the information contained in this book can be relevant to heterosexual men as well.

Although my previous book, *A Gay Man's Guide to Prostate Cancer*, was published in 2005, most of the essays were written between 2003 and 2004. Much has changed in the world of prostate cancer since then. Early diagnosis has geometrically increased and new procedures have followed. When the book was first published, Viagra, Cialis, and Levitra had just come on the market. Laparoscopic surgery was in its infancy, and watchful waiting (active surveillance) was not typically recommended. Now the latter is a seriously considered option. As noted in the previous work, my co-editor and I could find only one openly gay urologist. Now I am aware of many others.

In the first book, most of the men writing about their experiences were barely six months out of diagnosis and/or treatment. The current book is not about describing where they are now. In fact, the vast majority of the experiential writers are new to this book and they have been diagnosed with and/or treated for prostate cancer some time ago. *What Every Gay Man Needs to Know about Prostate Cancer* addresses issues and experiences that were not mentioned in the previous volume. For example, what it is like to have a penile implant, to inject oneself with a needle to get an erection, to ejaculate urine where semen used to be, to go through the details of an open radical prostatectomy vs. the experience of robotic laparoscopic surgery, to choose watchful waiting as a treatment option, to live with the effects of hormone treatment, or to experience advanced cancer as a middle-aged gay man. With the permission of the authors, two essays from the previous publication are included in this volume with up-to-date additions from each author. In order to expand on the issues noted, among others, I am pleased to present *What Every Gay Man Needs to Know about Prostate Cancer*.

This book is divided into two sections: the

professional and the experiential. Part of the process of coping with any adversity life throws one's way begins with the acquisition of information about the problem with which one is dealing. Lack of knowledge is a great hindrance to coping effectively with any trauma. It is hoped that this book will help expand the reader's knowledge regarding prostate cancer as it affects gay men. Thus, the first section is devoted to expanding that knowledge base for gay men with PCa and for those who love and care for them, as well as for those who treat them. You may come across many terms and references with which you may not be familiar. The glossary at the back of the book explains most of the terms used in this book.

In the first essay presented in the professional section, Dr. Lara Descartes et al. discuss gay men's knowledge of PCa and the male reproductive anatomy in general; the authors differentiate the degree of accurate information possessed by gay men as it correlates with socio-economic status and ethnicity. They write also of the paucity of information available to men of color and male-to-female (MTF) transgender people. The essay that follows, by Drs. Franklin Lowe and Vincent Santillo, is an attempt to further fill the gap in that knowledge by bringing us up-to-date information regarding the effects of the various treatments for PCa on quality-of-life issues.

The next professional essay deals with how to cope with erectile dysfunction (ED). Following a discussion of the male sexual system, Dr. Raanan Tal presents a very readable and comprehensive view of how the major treatments available for prostate cancer affect sexual functioning. He also writes, in a very hopeful manner, about how gay men may cope with and treat ED. As a corollary, Dr. Tal teams up with Dr. Steven Goldstone in the next essay to discuss, in particular, issues concerning sexual activity following prostate cancer treatment. Then Dr. Matthew Lemer discusses prostatic health and coping with urinary incontinence that may result from the treatment of PCa, with a particular emphasis on gay men's issues regarding this vexing problem. The professional section continues with Drs. Matthew Wosnitzer and Franklin Lowe's look at HIV status and its relationship to prostate cancer diagnosis and treatment in the era of highly-active antiretroviral treatment (HAART).

Transitioning to a more psychological perspective, Darryl Mitteldorf, a therapist specializing in treating men with cancer, describes pertinent issues in the psychotherapy of gay men who have been recently diagnosed with prostate cancer regarding coming out to their doctors. He also presents helpful suggestions for health care professionals in order to make it easier for gay men to feel safe enough to be open with them. Mitteldorf contributes a second essay about things he has learned from working with gay men who have prostate cancer, in support groups and individually (in person and online). Next, speaking from his experience as a straight urologist treating gay men with prostate cancer, Dr. Franklin Lowe addresses the patient and physician regarding his recommendations for both as they interact in the course of the diagnosis and treatment of prostate cancer.

The second section of book speaks from a more experiential, psychological, and practical vantage point. It is comprised of writing by gay men who have been struggling with PCa themselves. They write of their experience, sharing their thoughts and feelings in open, heartfelt, and often very moving ways: Each man facing the anxiety of being diagnosed, having to make a treatment decision, and dealing with the consequences of those decisions in his own particular way. Most of these authors have had some form of aggressive treatment for their prostate cancer; only one has not. The reader will note that most of the gay men writing about their experiences are from the New York City area; that is because they were

8

participants in a gay group that I facilitated under the auspices of Malecare, Inc.

The experiential section begins with "Mark Red" being diagnosed with PCa and selecting watchful waiting/active surveillance as his treatment choice in the midst of dealing with his sexual compulsivity. Next, John Dalzell presents his very analytical method of making a decision about which treatment he considered best for himself. He then goes on to report how, despite his carefully calculated protocol, he still had to deal with all the anxieties and concerns about being diagnosed with and treated for PCa. This is followed by an essay by Milton Sonday, who describes his rather anxiety-free experience of accepting what the doctor ordered and feeling very comfortable with that choice. In addition to providing an easily understood treatise on male sexual anatomy and how it works, he presents the reader with things he wished he knew about and had been prepared for as he coped with the treatment of and recovery from a radical prostatectomy. In a similar vein, "Paul Jarod" chronicles his journey from diagnosis to treatment to recovery, sharing his feelings, and giving tips on what to expect and look for before and after any kind of invasive procedure, prostatectomy or otherwise. He also suggests ways a gay man might cope with sexual encounters following surgery.

Two essays discuss the experience of robotic laparoscopic surgery. The first essay, by Gil Tunnell, details his coping strategies for dealing with the myriad of feelings accompanying the diagnosis and treatment of PCa. He discusses coping with anxiety, depression, denial, anger, and uncertainty. "James Larsen," in a second essay regarding robotic laparoscopic surgery, describes in very candid and down-to-earth terms how, as a gay man in his early forties, he learned to deal with the particular side effects of surgery that he experienced. He is quite candid about how he has been coping with ejaculating urine where

9

he used to shoot semen.

In an updated version of his essay in *A Gay Man's Guide to Prostate Cancer*, Lidell Jackson, a self-proclaimed sex-positive gay man, compares his struggle with HIV to his experience of being diagnosed and treated for prostate cancer. As an African-American, he raises the awareness flag to black men who are at greater risk of the disease and calls special attention to the role of testosterone among gay men and its impact on prostate cancer. In an updated version of his essay from the same book, Roberto Martinez, a self-described sexually active Latino gay man, reveals how the radical prostatectomy he underwent affected his thoughts and feelings, and especially his behavior, regarding his own sexuality. He relates how the physical changes he experienced engendered emotional changes in his own struggles concerning sex with partners and with masturbation.

Joe Davenport and John Frank have each contributed essays about their physical, psychological, and emotional reactions to discovering that, following surgery, they were each unable to get erections. They speak openly about how much an erect penis has defined them as gay men, especially as sexually active gay men. After the many trials and tribulations of trying various treatments to correct their erectile dysfunction, both men opted to have penile implants. Joe's verdict on his new apparatus is still up in the air. Frank, on the other hand, describes feeling very happy with his ability to get an erection at will. These stories bring home, once again, how varying an individual's physical and emotional reactions to treatment choices and outcomes can be.

As a relatively young, sexually active gay man, "Charles Godfry" underwent an open radical prostatectomy. Then his cancer returned several years later. He writes honestly about his struggle with advanced cancer, his having ultimately undergone hormonal treatment, external beam radiation, and cryotherapy; he writes about his depression and his attempt to stay hopeful and connected as well as sexual.

The book concludes with an updated glossary of technical terms, an appendix of references relating to each essay respectively, and a list of resources for those seeking further information and/or looking to speak with other gay men who are either going through or have been through what the reader may be experiencing.

It becomes very apparent to any man diagnosed with prostate cancer that there are no clear-cut answers or solutions to the issues that confront him. Each man must make his own decision regarding what to do and how to cope with that decision. It has been my experience that ultimately each man makes the decision that is right for him and then must learn to adjust to the new reality that follows. Being gay only exacerbates and complicates the many difficulties and uncertainties facing men diagnosed with PCa for many of the reasons articulated in this book.

It is hoped that the contributions made herein will help inform, clarify, and validate many of the experiences facing gay men so that they and their loved ones may make better-informed decisions, be aware of what may follow from these decisions, and how to better cope with whatever comes their way as a result of struggling with prostate cancer. It is also hoped that What Every Gay Man Needs to Know about Prostate Cancer will inform and help the professional (whether urologist, oncologist, mental health practitioner, or primary care physician) working with gay men diagnosed with and/or treated for prostate cancer so that he/she may be clearer about what technical, emotional, physical, and psychological issues each man may be dealing with, and how to validate and guide them as they struggle through the vicissitudes of coping with prostate cancer.

Today we are hearing about new drugs that deal with

advanced prostate cancer, such as Provenge (sipuleucel-T) and Abiratone (Zytiga). Also getting some attention is the controversial use of the drug Dutasteride, which may slow or stop tumors. However, there seems to be a downside to using this drug; it may fuel the growth of more dangerous prostate cancers. Much more research is needed to resolve this controversy. In addition, there is preliminary news about tests that could lead to earlier detection of PCa. Some of these tests involve urine; others evaluate blood. We may be moving toward a time when it will be possible to clearly differentiate potentially-lethal cancers from those that are not life threatening.

Recently, as many may have heard or read, the United States Preventive Services Task Force has come out against routine PSA blood tests for the screening of prostate cancer. They concluded that based on PSA diagnosis there have been too many unnecessary treatments with their consequent side effects to justify testing being done routinely. While their recommendations are not binding, their guidelines are usually followed by most physicians. Another concern is that insurance companies may use these guidelines to refuse payment for these very expensive tests.

The PSA test has its limitations, but when used correctly it allows urologists and other physicians to identify those men needing a biopsy. It is up to the treating physician to be more aware of those men who need to be treated and those who do not.

Like many other issues surrounding prostate cancer, there are no simple answers. The debate and controversy will continue. One thing seems clear: According to the urologists with whom I have spoken, there has been a decrease in the number of deaths due to prostate cancer since PSA testing began.

So, in the light of all the uncertainly and controversy surrounding prostate cancer, I am nevertheless delighted to present this book with the conviction that it will assist gay men, their loved ones, and those who treat them to better understand the particular concerns of the gay man navigating the very confusing labyrinth surrounding the diagnosis and treatment of prostate cancer.

Part One

Professional Section

Gay Men's Knowledge of Prostate Cancer

Lara Descartes, PhD, Marysol Asencio, DrPH, Thomas O. Blank, PhD, and
Ashley Crawford, MA

Prostate cancer is the most common male cancer, and it is also the most age-related. Men over the age of sixty have a greater than one-in-six chance of a prostate cancer diagnosis—all older men have to consider at least the prospect of dealing with prostate cancer. Increased screening with prostate specific antigen (PSA) has resulted in some men in their forties and fifties dealing directly with prostate cancer. Middle-aged men thus also should attend to and know about the realities of prostate cancer. There is a need to educate younger as well as older men about this important health concern. Those affected by prostate cancer also can be of any sexual orientation. Yet, gay couples may be more likely than heterosexual couples to experience prostate cancer within their intimate relationships—gay male couples are comprised of two men. Santillo & Lowe (2005) reported that for a gay couple "there is a 28% chance that one partner will be diagnosed with prostate cancer over their lifetime and a 3% chance that both partners will be diagnosed."

Until very recently, however, there was no research on prostate cancer conducted specifically with gay men. The necessity and importance of this research is self-evident given the number of gay men that may be affected by prostate cancer. More information is needed to understand gay and bisexual men's knowledge about prostate cancer, the context in which they receive medical care, and their need for social support. This information will help gay men cope with both the physical implications and emotional demands should they be faced with a cancer diagnosis and will help medical staff create an inclusive environment for providing supportive health care to all of their patients, regardless of sexual orientation.

Prostate cancer usually progresses slowly. This means that not only are many older men diagnosed with prostate cancer, but those who are diagnosed and treated at younger ages may live a significant portion of their adult lives as prostate cancer survivors. Part of prostate cancer's significance to men and their partners is the dramatic impact the treatments usually have upon their bodies, their sexuality, and their sense of masculinity. Common treatments include surgery, radiation, and hormonal ablation; all have side effects that may include erectile difficulties, incontinence, penile shrinkage, retrograde ejaculation, and bowel and rectal irritation. Many quantitative studies have been published that document these factors and their relationship to men's quality-of-life. Several qualitative studies have detailed the impact of prostate cancer and its treatments on sexuality. These qualitative studies in particular have provided important windows into the struggles men who have had prostate cancer go through to try to re-establish or re-understand and reframe their sense of themselves as sexual beings after the assaults of the disease and, especially, the treatments.

Together, the many studies on post-treatment quality-of-life have resulted in considerable understanding of the impact of prostate cancer. However, there are still significant gaps in the literature. First, while the focus quite rightly is on the impacts felt by men who have had prostate cancer, there has been less attention to the knowledge and attitudes of middle-aged and older men who have not experienced prostate cancer directly. Still, such information can be extremely important for formulating policy and clinical advice vis-à-vis screening, treatment choices, and so forth. What men think about the prostate generally, and prostate cancer specifically, whether the physiology, etiology, and/or the imagined or projected impact of treatment on quality-of-life, may powerfully influence their choices and behaviors related to prostate health and prostate cancer. Their knowledge and attitudes also form the basis for communications within the community and with health providers, especially first-line primary care physicians and general urologists.

Since the early 1990s, some important work has been conducted, investigating men's knowledge of prostate cancer and, especially, perceived knowledge of risk and attitude toward screening. There is a clear consensus within these studies on two specific points. First, middle-aged and older men are not well informed about major aspects of prostate cancer and its treatments. Some men overestimate their risk, while others underestimate it; some react to the potential of prostate cancer to be lethal (that is, they assume it is always life-threatening) and others ignore the potential threat to life. Many underestimate the potential for deleterious side effects of treatment, which can have such large impact on men's health and well-being. As a result, when personally confronted with prostate cancer, they may feel pressured into making decisions more quickly and with less knowledge than would be optimal for them. Second, the lack of knowledge is especially apparent among low income and African-American men. A study by Deibert et al. (2007) showed that low-income and little formal education were associated with having little understanding of the disease in their sample of men with prostate cancer. Almost every study that has considered race and ethnicity has found African-American men to have low levels of knowledge in general about prostate cancer, despite their heightened potential for it (especially its lethal form). A 2009 study by Kilbridge et al. presents a particularly distressing picture of African-American men's knowledge of the anatomy affected by prostate cancer treatments (prostate, bowels, bladder) and common terms used in patient literature and by health professionals relevant to prostate cancer (impotent, erection, rectal urgency, bowel function, among others.)

While critically important, most of these studies tapped into very specific aspects of prostate cancer (usually perceived risk, and in some cases, attitudes toward screening and intentions to undergo screening). The degree to which that lack of knowledge is more broadly related to prostate health, the role of the prostate in sexual function, and the nature of prostate cancer treatments are still unclear, as is the specific question of gay men's awareness of these issues. Some might presuppose that gay men are more sophisticated about sexual knowledge than the general male population and that they might know more about the prostate as it can be pleasurably stimulated during anal intercourse, a form of sexual expression stereotyped as being associated with gay sexuality. However, the little data there are suggest that gay and bisexual men are as lacking in pertinent knowledge as heterosexual men. One study interviewed health care providers who worked with gay, bisexual, and transsexual (GBT) men. They reported a lack of clarity regarding the men's knowledge of the characteristics of anal cancer and screening and treatment choices similar to those found in studies of prostate cancer with a non-gay population.

There is little work on how racial/ethnic identity might shape gay men's awareness of prostate-health issues. One exception is a study by Heslin, Gore, King, and Fox (2008) that explored how screening for prostate cancer related to race and sexual orientation. The researchers found that, although gay men in general did not differ from the heterosexual-identified population, African-American gay men were considerably less likely than other gay men and African-American heterosexuals to obtain prostate cancer screenings. More attention should be focused on minority racial/ethnic groups, including Spanish-speaking Latinos, who are not included in most studies.

Because of these factors and the prevalence of prostate cancer, it is important that medical providers address the specific needs of subpopulations of men who may be dealing with prostate cancer, including gay, bisexual men, and transgendered male-to-female (MTF) people. However, the medical system may not recognize the existence, needs, and concerns of gay, bisexual, and MTF people. There have been severe criticisms of the health care system as heterosexist and homophobic. As such, it may render gay men and their partners invisible. Moreover, gay men may have had negative experiences related to their sexual orientation in the clinical encounter or medical care setting due to provider bias and/or discrimination in access to high-quality health insurance. These experiences, or fear of such experiences, may lead gay patients to withhold personal information about their sexual orientation, sexual practices, and other factors. This may lead to significant delays in obtaining early screening and needed health care, jeopardizing successful treatment options and survival rates. Unfortunately, there is limited training on gay and bisexual men's lives in medical schools.

Finally, gay, bisexual, and MTF folks who find themselves facing a prostate cancer diagnosis need to think about what sources of support are available to them. Some men attend self-help groups upon diagnosis in order to share information and talk with others in the same situation. These groups, however, tend to have a hetero-normative bias and to assume that men's wives are their most important source of support. How might gay and bisexual men feel about attending such support groups?

In our study we address some of these gaps in the

literature by using data from five focus groups to examine gay men's knowledge of the prostate, prostate screenings, and prostate cancer risk factors and treatments. The research addresses these orienting questions: What is the men's knowledge about the prostate, including prostate cancer, risk factors, screenings, and treatment? How might sexual identity connect to gay men's experiences in the health care system and their perceived sources of information and support in the event of prostate cancer?

We gathered data on men's knowledge of prostate cancer and related issues through focus groups. These were an ideal format in which to hear the men's ideas and concerns, expressed in their own words. Focus groups enable participants to tell their own stories, hear what others have to say, and build upon and respond to others' words.

Our research team designed the focus group guide together, utilizing our individual backgrounds in health research, sexuality research, and qualitative research. Our initial literature review, including the first-person accounts of gay prostate cancer survivors included in A Gay Man's Guide to Prostate Cancer, also informed our question design.

An informational component was included in our procedure. We realized that the men would not have uniform or necessarily accurate knowledge of the prostate and our other themes of interest. After we led the men in an initial discussion of these topics to ascertain extent of their knowledge, the third author used a diagram to show the men where the prostate is located and discussed the basic facts of screening, prostate cancer, its treatments, and their side effects. The men were eager for this knowledge, and seemed to greatly appreciate access to reliable, clear information.

The men also completed a demographic questionnaire before the focus groups began. They filled out information including age, race, health insurance status, partnered status, preferred types of sexual activity, and so forth. They then completed a scale measuring their perceived knowledge about the prostate and prostate health.

This study was conducted in Hartford, Connecticut, a small northeastern city with a significant Latino and African-American/black population. There are not that many venues for gay life in the community. There are a few small bars and a few LGBT organizations. At the time of this study, the gay and lesbian community center had closed. There was no organization actively addressing the needs of older gay men. We recruited our study members through flyers at the community organizations that did have programming directed at gay men, and the local Pride celebration. We also placed postings on relevant listservs and enlisted local community organizers to help recruit participants. Our flyers and postings asked for "gay men interested in a study on prostate health issues." Our diverse recruitment locations and methods gave us a sample with a range of socioeconomic backgrounds and a significant number of Latino and black participants. This essay uses the term "black" to refer to men of African descent, whether African-American or Caribbean. The term "Latino" is also an umbrella term, referring to men from Puerto Rican, Mexican, and Latin American backgrounds.

We had a total of thirty-six participants in our five focus groups. Their average age was forty-nine years old, and their average education was "some college." One focus group was entirely composed of Spanish-speaking Latino men and was conducted in Spanish. Another group was entirely black men. The remaining groups were racially/ethnically mixed, but primarily non-Latino white. Although our recruitment was aimed at gay men, a number of bisexual men chose to participate, as did one male-to-female transsexual. Expecting only gay-identified men, we did not include a question on our demographic questionnaire specifically about sexual identity, and we thus are unaware of exactly how many men identified as gay vs. bisexual or transgender. The men's occupations varied greatly: from clerical and non-skilled labor to professional (e.g., lawyer, teacher). Six men identified themselves as disabled. Almost all of the participants had some form of health insurance, roughly equally divided between private employer-paid, Medicaid, and Medicare.

Half of the men were currently partnered. Thirty of the men had had sex in the past six months. Reporting on the previous year, 26% stated they had had zero male sexual partners, 39% one, and the rest from two to five; one participant had twenty. Types of sexual activities ranged broadly: Most men participated in multiple forms of sexual expression, for example participating in oral sex, anal sex, and so forth. Considering "importance of sex," the men were almost equally divided in rating it as important, not important, or in between.

Four of the five focus groups were moderated by the third author of this study. A fifth, a Spanish-speaking group of mixed Latino ethnicities, was moderated by the second author, who is a bilingual/bicultural Latina researcher. She took detailed notes during all five focus groups on content and group dynamics. All participants were provided with informed consent and all the procedures and materials utilized in this study were approved by the University of Connecticut's Institutional Review Board. After they were provided with informed consent, the men were remunerated with forty dollars. They were told that they could leave the group any time they wished. The men who chose to participate stayed the length of the discussion; only one who began needed to leave early.

The notes were commented upon and discussed by the research team after each focus group. The focus groups were subsequently transcribed. The notes and transcriptions were used by the authors to conduct thematic analyses, identifying group-level trends and subgroup or individual issues that came up in the group discussions.

Our data confirm prior studies conducted with presumptively heterosexual populations in depicting a striking lack of knowledge among men regarding their prostates, potential prostate problems, and prostate cancer screening. Variations in race/ethnicity, socioeconomic status, and age corresponded to different levels of knowledge. We also address how the men discussed access to medical care, specifically as related to their sexual identities, and the possibilities of obtaining support should they be diagnosed with prostate cancer.

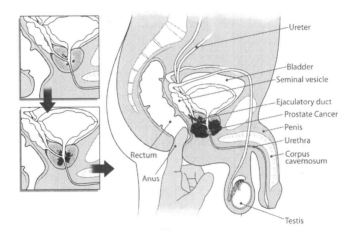

The Prostate and Prostate Exams

The men who participated in the focus groups showed widely varying levels of understanding about their bodies, especially their prostates. Most evinced little and/or faulty knowledge about issues related to the prostate. Many were unaware not only of the prostate's function, but of its location. They did know it was in the lower part of the body, and often placed it near either the colon or anus. This exchange, for example, was heard in one group:

"I think it's somewhere around . . . somewhere between your legs somewhere."

"Somewhere up in the bowels."

"I believe near the anus. It's up around there."

"No, it's not!"

"It's up around there."

Similarly, someone in another group, when asked by the moderator where the prostate is, replied, "Your rectum."

"Under your scrotum."

"Oh yeah, behind it or something?"

Most were similarly unaware of the prostate's role in making semen, postulating that its function had something to do with urination, penile erection, or digestion. Some were unaware that it was a specifically male organ—"Do only men have prostates?" The men showed similarly low levels of knowledge when discussing what could go wrong with the prostate; one used the word "hernia" to describe potential problems, for example. Many confused issues of enlargement vs. cancer. The levels of knowledge directly corresponded to the men's racial/ethnic backgrounds and perceived socio-economic status (SES): Those who were minorities, non-English speakers, and those who seemed to have lower SES (and reported being on Medicaid) were less likely to have accurate knowledge of any of the discussed topics.

The lack of general knowledge about the prostate compromised other types of information, such as awareness about prostate screening. The confusion about the location and function of the prostate led some to assume that the colonoscopy exam was also a prostate exam since it was perceived as an "anal exam." For example, one man stated that he had "a 'prostate' done. That is a pain. They put a tube in there and they put you to sleep." Another man, African-American, related: "I know very little about

26

[prostate cancer], anything at all. There's cancer somewhere…what I think is cancer somewhere about my colon in my body. I did have it tested. And my prostate was swollen. And they called it early stages. What I don't know if it's going to come back. I did go on medication."

Further probing by the researchers indicated this was not early stage prostate cancer but probably an enlarged prostate.

A number of participants assumed that if their colonoscopy exam showed no problems, which meant they had no prostate problems.

Several men were unsure about whether they had indeed received a prostate screening from their physicians. Very few had heard of PSA tests. More knew about the digital rectal exam, and many had experienced at least one. However, many did not know why they were receiving it or even that it was a prostate exam. One man asked if physicians administering the digital rectal exam would be able to tell if he were gay. Other comments we heard included "When I was younger, I always wondered what they were doing" and "I never knew why he was putting his finger in." A few, in contrast, made aware of prostate cancer through televised public awareness campaigns, had requested and received a screening from their physicians.

Discussions of the digital rectal exam in particular provided a focus for the men's humor. One Latino man reported, for example, to great group hilarity, that he and his partner performed the exam on each other annually. A man in a different focus group reported that his doctor had small hands, so the exams were always painless, likewise receiving a great deal of laughter. Yet another chuckled as he related how, while undergoing the digital rectal exam, he'd told his doctor to buy him dinner first. The men did acknowledge discomfort around the intimate nature of this particular screening. One stated that his physician, with whom he was friendly, seemed uncomfortable when he asked for the exam, and noted that he was uncomfortable himself due to their personal relationship. Eventually the physician brought a female clinician into the office to perform the procedure. These various stories likely point to the men's awareness of the obvious linkages to be made between a penetrative anal exam and anal sex, as well as the stereotypes with which heterosexuals might frame gay men's experiences in receiving such exams.

Participants' age also played a role in their overall knowledge. A few of the older participants had begun having problems with their prostates. Thus, they, through their clinicians, were being educated about certain aspects of prostate anatomy and problems. Even they, however, had gaps in their knowledge, which may also have been related to their SES and the quality of the clinical care they were receiving.

Prostate Cancer Risk Factors and Treatment

When the focus groups discussed risk factors for prostate cancer, a few suggested that some men are at higher risk because of their genetics: "I believe if someone down the line in your family had it, then it could be passed down from generation to generation. I don't know if that's true but that's what I believe." Some were not so sure: "It's not something that's hereditary, is it?" A few suggested that hormone imbalances could explain why a man would get prostate cancer. Some related risk to a man's personal health history, such as whether he smoked or ate meat, and/or whether he had high levels of stress. A few black men added that they understood their race placed them at higher risk for prostate cancer, which they related to stress and poor quality health care: "The lack of health care in the black community . . . plays a lot in whether [black men] get checked early or get diagnosed really late." "It can be a lot of stress levels too . . . what we deal with every day being black." As with basic knowledge of the prostate and prostate exams, those men who were older and had begun to encounter prostate issues were the most likely to be informed about risk.

One topic the men were very unclear on (as indeed are researchers) and curious about was whether one's risk for contracting prostate cancer had anything to do with being the receptive partner in anal sex. We noticed that the focus groups debated as to whether being the receptive partner in anal sex and the resultant stimulation of the prostate might be preventative of prostate cancer or causative.

A significant majority of the participants were unaware or unsure about the available treatment options should they get prostate cancer, and so tended to discuss the topic using their overall knowledge of cancer rather than knowledge about prostate cancer specifically (this likely holds true for their discussion of risk factors as well). For example, almost all mentioned chemotherapy, which is not commonly used to treat prostate cancer. They also mentioned surgery and/or radiation treatments, which indeed are used to treat prostate cancer. However, many were surprised to hear about androgen deprivation therapy as a treatment, which is regularly used in cases of advanced prostate cancer.

Latino participants were more likely than non-Latino men to suggest non-traditional healing and spiritually-focused means as possible treatments, in addition to radiation and chemotherapy. As one man put it, "When someone doesn't have faith they don't have hope. Hope for me is the motive for fighting, it is the key, it is a rock in your life. From there you can fight. If you have faith, you believe. Faith helps you."

As reported elsewhere, we were surprised to find that the participants were almost completely unaware of the potential side effects of treatment options for prostate cancer. These of course can quite dramatically affect daily life and sexuality, with different treatments potentially resulting in urinary incontinence, erectile difficulties, penile shrinkage, and bowel irritation, as examples. Upon learning of the potential side effects, the men agreed that these should be considered when deciding upon treatment options. If one preferred to be anally receptive, for instance, treatment options that might irritate the bowel might best be avoided.

Concerns About and Experiences with the Medical System

Many focus group participants, regardless of their racial/ethnic or socioeconomic background, stated that finding a trustworthy health care provider was of utmost importance for successful aging, including dealing with any potential problems with the prostate and sexuality. Also noted as important was the ability to communicate with their health care provider and, by some, to be open about their sexuality. Yet, the majority also stated that they were not out to their doctors. Some presumed their doctors already knew their sexual orientation, and others questioned why such a thing would be relevant to the doctor-patient relationship. Typical comments were that coming out to one's provider would be "immaterial" or that "you have to keep it [being gay] quiet." Some men worried that physicians would think they had AIDS if they reported they were gay. One man reported that, "I wouldn't say anything because I am there to get help. I am not here for you to find out about my sexual life." The men noted sexuality and sexual issues aren't often discussed by medical care providers.

The men generally expressed that they themselves currently had good doctors who were receptive to their needs and communicated well, a number reported that they had experienced homophobic medical care. Unfortunately, many accepted that homophobia was a reality for gay men and felt it was pervasive throughout the medical community. A few men related being verbally harassed and suffering poor medical care when their physicians found out they were gay. One Latino man said, "I would enter [my doctor's] office and it seemed like it was an insult to him that he saw me. And that happened after I told him that I am gay. While I did not tell him I am gay, he got along well with me . . . [In general], if they know I am gay, they'll treat me last." One man reported suffering a rough and insensitive digital rectal exam, which he attributed to the doctor being aware that he was gay and wanting to make sure he did not enjoy the exam. This issue of enjoying the exam "too much" due to one's gay or bisexual identity arose several times in the focus groups.

Obtaining decent health insurance was a priority for many focus group participants. For those who did have health insurance, many had not considered what it might or might not cover should they be diagnosed with prostate cancer. A majority of participants expressed fears about losing coverage and not having access to necessary care. In terms of seeking care should they receive a prostate cancer diagnosis, many of the men said they would have to first find out what types of treatment their insurance would cover. Men who received state-funded insurance all agreed that it was quite inadequate. The amount of red tape necessary to obtain treatment was so daunting that many men simply gave up if they needed something. Most argued in favor of nationalized health insurance and increased prevention screening as alternative, long-term solutions to the problems of finding competent care.

Many of the men believed that access to the best medical care requires a great deal of money and a detailed knowledge of the health care system (as two men said, "medical care is based on your money" and "if you don't have the money, you're not going to get the proper care").

Further, they believed that a higher-priced doctor might not want to treat some groups, such as current or ex-drug users. With this in mind, those participants who did or had used drugs felt that should they need health care, their choices might be rather limited. On the other hand, several seemed to have an unrealistic idea of access to medical care, such as when men who had relatively minimal state-financed insurance said they would "obviously pick out the best physician that has a good track record in treating prostate cancer" if they were to be diagnosed.

Finally, HIV is a prominent health concern in the gay male community. Its prevention and treatment were acknowledged in focus groups as overshadowing any concerns about prostate health. Men in the Latino group suggested that "everything is geared towards HIV/AIDS in the gay community" and therefore discussion surrounding prostate cancer is not prominent; thus gay men are not as educated about it as they are about HIV. The few men who were HIV-positive in the focus groups discussed how their HIV specialists were not concerned about any health problem that they saw as unrelated to their HIV: "If it is not AIDS-related, then don't bother." Thus, they felt they would have to move outside these providers to treat non-HIV related health problems: "I do not think our HIV doctor ever tested [my partner and me] for prostate cancer . . . he is an AIDS specialist. Unless it is proven to be AIDS-related, he is going to refer you to someone else." These men also complained that physicians wouldn't listen to them about non-HIV concerns, such as prostate issues, because of an attitude of "You are going to die anyway. Why waste our time with you?" As another man put it, "If you have AIDS, they don't care."

Concerns about Support Groups

Focus group participants talked about the problems of

living in a homophobic society, including being rejected by society, mental health issues related to experiencing discrimination, and assumptions that illnesses were signs of punishment from God. They recognized that prostate cancer could be a serious issue, especially in combination with such homophobic attitudes, and that they would need support should they be diagnosed with prostate cancer. Most stated they would seek support from their partners, friends, or immediate family. The Latino group added that they would seek spiritual counseling. Some of the men also expressed interest in joining support groups, which are a common source of information and support for prostate cancer survivors and their partners.

Many of the men stated at first that they did not care whether such a group's membership was primarily gay or heterosexual. They felt that prostate cancer was a "man's issue" as opposed to a "gay issue." They argued that all men can get prostate cancer, and thus sexuality would not be relevant to the information and aid to be had from joining a support group. One Latino participant said, "[Heterosexuals] carry the same [set of genitals] that I carry. They use it differently, but it is the same biological system." As another man put it, "It is the prostate. It doesn't care if you are gay or straight, black or white or yellow."

Some men, however, expressed a desire for gay-only support groups: "I guess a gay support group would feel more comfortable because if you are gay you are quote, unquote, labeled. You know what I mean? So for me, a gay support group would be more comfortable." Another man agreed, adding that for another issue, "I went to a group of straight men that was a men's group. It was very difficult because I thought I was more sensitive than most of them. I don't know; it was just different. It was very difficult for me in the straight group. I wasn't comfortable sharing my personal feelings when they were sharing about their wives." Another added, "Straight men don't know the difference of gay sex."

Even men who initially thought they wouldn't care whether a prostate cancer support group was gay or not changed their perspectives when the moderator asked how they might feel discussing sexuality issues in a non-gay group. The men were surprised such issues might come up. The moderator mentioned that some men might discuss their difficulties in having sex with their wives, as an example. This changed our participants' outlook. They indicated that they were not interested in hearing about heterosexual men's sexual problems, and would not be comfortable discussing their own sexual concerns in such an environment. As one man put it, "I think things would be discussed in [a support group] that people would really shy away from . . . So yeah, I think it would be important if they had gay-specific support groups." And when the men learned that heterosexual men's wives might be present at the group discussions, they agreed that that would make it awkward to discuss openly their sexuality and sexual dysfunction. Many of the African-American men stated that it would be difficult for them to discuss any sexual dysfunction in the first place, regardless of who might be in the group. They seemed to be expressing a sense that African-American men are "supposed to be" virile and that black men feel they need to present a highly masculine posture. No alternative representations of black masculinity were raised by the participants.

The men thus agreed that gay-only support groups would be most beneficial for discussing specifically sexual concerns, though they indicated they would attend mixed support groups to learn about treatment options. Racial/ethnic minority participants stated that having minority-only support groups would be more beneficial for them. Many felt that they shared the same issues as other gay men with access to health care, but in addition to homophobia they had to deal with racism and xenophobia.

34

As one participant put it, "Information has to be out there that's relevant, you know. I'm a gay black man and I'm not alone." Many participants in the Spanish-speaking Latino gay male group mentioned that Spanish-speaking groups were of utmost concern, as there are many who might wish to seek medical treatment but would not because of language barriers.

Conclusions

Our research corroborates previous studies indicating that middle-aged and older men are not knowledgeable about prostate health and prostate cancer, while adding that this lack of knowledge extends to basic physiological understanding on the one side, and, due to side effects of treatments, social and relationship impacts on the other. It also forcefully verifies the consistent findings that degree of knowledge cleaves dramatically along racial/ethnic, SES, and other demographic factors.

Racial/ethnic minority men in our study reported needing targeted campaigns about prostate cancer, screening, and treatment, a recommendation that has support in the literature. A 2003 study, for example, discussed differences between African-American and Latino men in overall life concerns, health concerns, and preferred modes of learning about prostate cancer. A number of the African-American participants in our study stated that they were afraid of negative diagnoses, however, and therefore might not seek screening at all. They argued that in general, the notion of "I don't want to know" pervades the African-American community.

On a more encouraging note, Wilkinson et al. (2003) found that a one-hour information session greatly enhanced the knowledge base of African-American men about the disease. A session that explicated physiological characteristics, treatment choices, potential psychological and social impacts, and decision aids in general, would be useful in helping gay and bisexual men, especially if it incorporated specific attention to the issues that are more specific to a sexual minority population. Such an educational measure appears both practical and likely to have a significant positive impact on the community.

A special note should be made of the specific concerns of MTF transsexuals, one of whom participated in a focus group as noted. She contended that many MTF people were unaware that they even had prostates, which are not removed even in those who have undergone sex reassignment genital surgery. In fact, a small number of cases of MTF transgender persons who have developed and been treated for prostate cancer have been reported in the medical literature. It thus seems safe to say that educational measures targeted toward sexual minority communities might do well to include the fact that MTF transsexuals still have their prostates, and thus should be aware of risk factors for prostate cancer.

Health care and insurance were matters of great concern to most of the men in our sample. Our work demonstrates the need for medical providers to be very clear in their descriptions of procedures, risk factors, treatments, and side effects, whether for prostate cancer or other medical conditions. The men in our sample, especially those from low SES and/or minority backgrounds, were quite confused as to why they had had digital rectal examinations, what a colonoscopy was and wasn't for, and so on. In addition, the men in our study who were HIV-positive pointed out problematic aspects in their experiences in the medical system. Health issues need to be more comprehensively addressed, so that HIV- positive individuals receive quality care for their HIV- and non-HIV-related conditions. Further, the concerns the men in our sample expressed about obtaining quality health insurance reinforce Ramchand and Fox's (2007) discussion of access issues. Gay men, especially those who are poor and/or of a racial minority, can face numerous obstacles in finding complete, quality health coverage.

Of great concern are several studies that found that gay men who had experienced prostate cancer report significant concerns and impacts related to their sexual identity and that their experience was made more difficult because of uneven or prejudiced medical care. While some of these issues are certainly shared with a wide range of men, some are quite distinctively connected to being gay, bisexual, or transgender. The words of the men in our sample clearly indicate that homophobia remains a problem in the medical field; and that health care providers need to be sensitive to the possibility that their patients are not heterosexual and aware of their own biases about sexual minorities. Beyond basic sensitivity, proactive measures could be taken to address gay and bisexual men's fears and perceptions of homophobia. If the assumption is made that some men will be concerned about disclosing their sexual identity, then efforts could be made to encourage openness in the medical encounter. Signs could be posted, or intake materials could include information that makes patients aware that the environment is an inclusive one.

It also seems apparent that, in the event of prostate cancer, men with non-majority sexual and racial/ethnic identities need groups that are specific to them. These gay and bisexual focus group participants indicated that they would be most comfortable discussing sexuality and relationship issues among men who share their sexual identity. Racial/ethnic minority men said likewise. In areas where there are many Latinos, for example, Spanish-language support groups should be made available, including Spanish-language gay men's groups.

The findings discussed here reveal questions about anal sex and its potential connection to prostate cancer, whether preventative or causative. The possibility that anal sex and prostate stimulation may contribute to the development (or not) of prostate cancer has not been thoroughly studied. If a relationship were to be determined, it would have dramatic implications for any man, of whatever sexual identity, that practices this form of sex.

Our research, like any small-scale project, is not necessarily generalizable. However, our focus groups illustrate the value of including men with minority sexual identities, minority racial/ethnic identities, and diverse socioeconomic statuses into research on the common male problem of prostate cancer. Especially given the current economic climate, in future studies researchers should consider different types of disadvantage and how they might compound each other: for example, individuals who have recently lost their jobs and who are now without health insurance, and how such factors might interact with the problems and challenges related to minority identity that we have explored here.

Quality-of-Life and Cancer Control after Prostate Cancer Treatment

Vincent M. Santillo, MD and Franklin C. Lowe, MD, MPH, FACS

In 2009, the American Cancer Society estimated that more than 192,000 men were diagnosed with prostate cancer and more than 27,000 died from this disease. While screening has uncovered more and more cases, the five-year survival rates from 1996 to 2004 were 98.9% for all stages of prostate cancer with a 100.0% five-year survival rate for local disease, but were only 31.7% if the patient presented with distant metastasis at diagnosis. Relative ten-year and fifteen-year survival is 93% and 79%, respectively. Prostate cancer incidence has been in flux over the past twenty years as the full impact of the introduction of screening with the prostate-specific antigen (PSA) blood test was felt. After increasing from 1995 to 2001, incidence rates of prostate cancer have been declining by 4.4% per year since 2001. Even with improvements in the death rate, prostate cancer remains the second leading cause of cancer mortality in men after lung cancer (American Cancer Society, 2009).

The average American man has a 15.8% chance of being diagnosed with prostate cancer over his lifetime. While that overall rate would be expected to be similar in gay men, the impact of a prostate cancer diagnosis and possible treatment on both parties involved in an intimate relationship can be significant. For a gay couple that means that there is a 26.6% chance that either they or their partner will be diagnosed with prostate cancer.

Quality-of-life issues include:

1) Freedom from biochemical recurrence (effective cancer control).
2) Recovery of erectile function.
3) Recovery of continence.

More broadly this concept could be applied to other prostate cancer treatment modalities that may differ in how they define recurrent disease, but can also have their success or failure evaluated by how well the patients do in terms of continence and erectile function in addition to effective cancer control.

Effective Cancer Control

Treatment options include: expectant management/ observation/watchful waiting, radical prostatectomy, external beam radiotherapy (EBRT), brachytherapy (radioactive seed implant treatment), combination EBRT and brachytherapy, cryotherapy, and androgen deprivation therapy (ADT). Since the advent of PSA screening, the majority of prostate cancers are localized (confined to the capsule of the prostate gland) at the time of diagnosis and the numbers of patients who have undergone treatment with radiation and surgery has increased dramatically. Due to a lack of randomized controlled trials comparing the effectiveness and side effects of the various treatment modalities for managing clinically localized prostate cancer, patients can find that the information they receive in terms of optimal treatment is different depending on the specialist whose advice is sought. Even with the uncertain benefits of treatment, less than 10% of men opt for watchful waiting/active surveillance/expectant management. Regardless of whether they were treated with prostatectomy, radiation therapy, or conservative/expectant management, studies have shown that most men have excellent ten-year prostate cancer-specific survival. The decision for the type of intervention should be driven by patient preference.

Recovery of Erectile Function

A 2008 study reported on men with previously untreated stage T1/T2 prostate cancer (see glossary), who had opted for active treatment: prostatectomy, brachytherapy, or EBRT. The group used patient- and partner-reported outcome measures to identify the determinants of health-related quality-of-life after treatment for prostate cancer as well as to measure the impact of the determinants on patient and spouse or partner satisfaction with the outcome of treatment. They evaluated 1,201 men and 625 partners (99% of whom were female). Those in the radiotherapy group had the greatest number of coexisting illnesses, the brachytherapy group was intermediate, and the prostatectomy group had the least. The radiotherapy group presented with the most severe cancer, the prostatectomy group was intermediate, and the brachytherapy group had the least severe disease.

The study found that each group experienced a decrease in sexual quality-of-life after treatment. As expected, those patients who underwent a nerve-sparing vs. a non-nerve-sparing prostatectomy had a better recovery of sexual quality-of-life. Among those patients opting for EBRT, supplementation with androgen deprivation therapy led to worse recovery of sexual quality-of-life. The authors found that older age, large prostate size, and a high pretreatment PSA score were all associated with a worse sexual quality-of-life as compared with baseline. At twelve months, partners felt distress related to the patient's erectile dysfunction in 44% of the patients in the prostatectomy group, 22% of those receiving radiotherapy, and 13% of those receiving brachytherapy.

The significant short-term and long-term erectile

dysfunction after prostatectomy has led to an increased focus on intra-operative and possible post-operative interventions to reduce its incidence. The importance of preserving the cavernous nerves was first described by Walsh et al. And modifications to surgical technique continue to improve outcomes as shown in a study by Masterson et al. They hypothesized that the use of Foley traction (see glossary) during prostatectomy was placing tension on the neurovascular bundle and leading to worse outcomes and found a 22% improvement in erectile recovery at six months in those who were operated on using a modified technique without Foley traction. Recent surgical advances such as laparoscopic and robotic surgery have had uncertain impacts on surgical outcomes.

More recently, investigators have been evaluating whether any post-operative therapy might improve the return of patient erectile function post-prostatectomy. Montorsi et al. (1997) provided early evidence of a possible benefit in a small group of thirty patients that were randomized to receive Caverject (Alprostadil) injections three times per week for twelve weeks versus patients who were observed without erectogenic treatment. Eight patients (67%) in the treated group reported the recovery of spontaneous erection sufficient for intercourse, compared with three (20%) in the observation group. While the study had issues, it served to alert the medical community that the traditional practice of waiting one year prior to evaluate erectile function post-prostatectomy may be too long because a window of opportunity might be missed without early penile rehabilitation.

Earlier studies by Mulhall et al. (2009), demonstrated the benefits of PDE5 inhibitors, like Viagra, when taken on demand, more recent work has focused on regular protocols that may be beneficial. The study shows that pharmacological intervention during the convalescent period can enhance the recovery of spontaneous erections and provide objective data and a protocol for the now common clinical practice of providing Viagra postoperatively for variable periods of time. Different results were seen by Montorsi et al.

The topic is an area of continued controversy. But Mulhall feels that, "There is a clear signal from the human literature supported by robust animal data that there is a value to pharmacologic penile rehabilitation." He argued for the role of pharmacological rehabilitation while research continues, in light of "the significant reduction in health-related quality-of-life associated with long-term ED." Morgentaler took a far more negative view of the evidence for penile rehabilitation saying, "It appears that the strongest reason to offer pills for penile rehabilitation is to give our patients the feeling that we are doing something to improve the probability of sexual recovery, banking on the powerful cultural mythology attached to these medications. Clinical norms should be established only where there is strong evidence and a solid mechanistic foundation. Penile rehabilitation has neither." The debate goes on.

Urinary Issues

In a 2008 study, Sanda et al. found that in patients having surgery, the incontinence was at its worse at two months post-surgery and then improved in most cases. Greater levels of incontinence were associated with older age, black race, and a high PSA score at diagnosis. Prostatectomy patients did experience improvements in urinary irritation and obstruction scores. Patients in the radiotherapy group found that their urinary symptoms had resolved at twelve months and were above baseline at twenty-four months. Of note, the patients in the brachytherapy group had significant worsening of urinary irritation or obstruction and incontinence. In terms of having moderate or worse distress from overall urinary

43

symptoms at one year post-treatment, 18% of the brachytherapy group was in that category, 11% of those in the radiotherapy, but only 7% of those in the prostatectomy group. At one year, 5% of partners of those in the prostatectomy or brachytherapy groups were bothered by the patient's incontinence. In terms of partners being bothered by obstructive urinary symptoms in the patient (e.g., urinary frequency), 7% of partners in the brachytherapy group vs. 3% in both the radiotherapy group and prostatectomy group were bothered.

A recent study assessed health-related quality-of-life outcomes for patients four years after treatment for localized prostate cancer. As noted in a study by Sanda et al., the urinary issues vary depending on the modality of therapy selected by the patient. In another study of 475 men, Gore et al. found that urinary incontinence was more common after prostatectomy than after brachytherapy or external beam radiation. Of interest, they found that, while improvements are seen in urinary function over a period more than twenty-four months post-prostatectomy, the likelihood of continued functional recovery of urinary function was low beyond thirty months, which can help guide the timing of secondary therapies for incontinence. Should dysfunction persist, possible clinical interventions include behavior modification, medication, urethral sling (see glossary), or an artificial sphincter.

It was also found that patients treated with either type of radiation therapy experienced minor impairments in urinary control as compared to radical prostatectomy (RP) patients. However, patients receiving radiation therapy experienced more urinary storage and voiding symptoms than prostatectomy patients. In terms of comparing the two radiation modalities, the authors found that those patients opting for brachytherapy had more urinary storage and voiding symptoms than either those treated with EBRT or RP. Brachytherapy was associated with a lower likelihood than RP of regaining a baseline American Urological Association Symptom Index (AUASI) score, which evaluates urinary storage and voiding symptoms. However, the probability of regaining baseline function improved over the forty-eight month study. Conversely, those patients who opted for EBRT demonstrated worsening AUASI scores over the forty-eight month study. Also with a strong impact on quality-of-life, authors found that patients who had either form of radiation therapy reported more bowel dysfunction than RP patients.

A 2009 study looked at the choice men make between an artificial urinary sphincter, the current gold standard, and a male sling for post-prostatectomy incontinence (PPI). In the absence of long-term data comparing the two treatments, they found that patients were most likely to follow their surgeon's advice in terms of appropriate PPI therapy. However, when men were offered a choice, the study participants favored using a sling, even with its lack of long-term data, vs. a mechanical device like an artificial sphincter. This desire to avoid a mechanical device is a motivating factor in those men who go against a surgeon's suggestion to have one implanted.

Conclusion

Series have been published in regards to various groups and their rates of success with quality-of-life outcomes in their patients. Eastham et al. (2008) have published a nomogram that estimates the preoperative likelihood of an optimal outcome after radical prostatectomy. As the increasing research on quality-of-life outcomes shows, urinary and erectile function as well as cancer control are key to patient quality-of-life and are important concerns when considering potential therapies and treatments for localized prostate cancer. However, men must remember that post-intervention urinary control and erectile function (after either brachytherapy or radiation therapy or surgery) are likely never to be as good as they were pre-intervention; this is an important consideration when determining whether to choose expectant management/observation as a management approach for prostate cancer.

Prostate Cancer and Sexual Dysfunction in Gay Men

Raanan Tal, MD

Prostate cancer, the second most common cancer among men, is a major health concern in the United States and around the world. According to the American Cancer Society data, it is estimated that in 2009, 192,280 men in the United States will be diagnosed with and 27,360 men will die of prostate cancer; that is 25% of all new cancer cases and 9% of all cancer related deaths, respectively. Currently, men often have periodical prostate specific antigen (PSA) blood tests and are diagnosed early, typically in the fifth, sixth, or seventh decade of their life. The vast majority, over 90% of men with prostate cancer, are diagnosed before the cancer has spread beyond the prostate gland itself; they have several effective treatment options and their chances of cure are excellent. It is estimated that about two million prostate cancer survivors are living in the United States (American Cancer Society, 2009). Combining this information with a rough and conservative estimate of the percentage of gay men in the general male population to be about 3 to 5%, we can estimate that 6,000 to 10,000 gay men are diagnosed with prostate cancer each year and that 60,000 to 100,000 gay prostate cancer survivors live among us, and many more gay men are sex partners of men who were diagnosed with prostate cancer. Despite these significant numbers of gay men whose life and sex life are possibly affected by prostate cancer, the medical literature does not address the gay population specifically. Thomas O. Blank spoke to this absence in an essay titled "Gay Men and Prostate Cancer: Invisible Diversity," which was published in the Journal of Clinical Oncology in 2005. He highlighted the fact that although there were more than 40,000 medical publications on prostate cancer management and outcomes, there were none directly addressing the gay population. This raises the question, whether prostate cancer management should be individualized by sexual orientation.

Management of prostate cancer may include careful monitoring without any active treatment (often called "active surveillance" or "watchful waiting"); surgery to remove the prostate (radical prostatectomy); prostate irradiation (radiotherapy); or hormonal medications aimed at reducing testosterone, the principal male hormone. Unfortunately, all prostate cancer management options are associated with changes in sexual function and have important implications regarding sexual activity. Obviously, men confront difficulties performing sexually during or immediately after treatment, but there are also long-term or permanent sexual function consequences that last long after men have completed their cancer treatment and are cured. Moreover, men, and not infrequently their partners, experience sex life alterations starting from initial stages of evaluation for prostate cancer and coping with the news of being diagnosed with prostate cancer, even before treatment options are discussed. In sexually active men and couples, any adverse change in sexual function may have important impact on general quality-of-life and sense of well-being.

Unfortunately, we do not have medical literature on gay sexual function outcomes after prostate cancer treatments. Most of the studies focus on erectile function in heterosexual men, where successful outcome is defined as being able to perform vaginal penetration (Tal, 2009). This definition is irrelevant when it comes to gay sex. Another example of the obstacles in applying information from the straight medical literature to the gay population is radiation treatment. Although among the known side effects of radiation treatment for prostate cancer are anal pain, discomfort, and mucus discharge, the impact of these side effects of radiation on sexual function have never been studied. In this essay I combine the current medical knowledge and my experience working with patients, both gay and straight, to delineate the changes in sexual function that pertain to gay men.

Sexual performance problems, commonly referred to as "sexual dysfunction" in the medical literature, include various aspects of sexual activity among which are sexual drive and interest ("libido"), erection quality, the nature of ejaculation, orgasm intensity, and even changes in the length, girth, and shape of the penis. Sexual function of gay men may also include the ability to engage in and enjoy receptive anal sex. Some of these changes are psychologically based while others are related to changes that one's body undergoes with cancer treatments. For most men, if not all, the change in their sex life is a combination of psychological and biological factors. Some of these changes are unavoidable, but commonly there are various treatment options that can minimize the adverse impact of prostate cancer and its treatment on one's sexuality. Not infrequently men inquire about the expected impact of prostate cancer and its treatment on their sex life even before they receive any treatment. Some men seek sexual health treatment only months or even years after they have completed their prostate cancer treatment, and they are frustrated with their inability to recover their sex life. My philosophy is that getting the information early is the best strategy; it allows one to educate himself, his friends, family, and sexual partners. It also gives the man time to consider the options carefully before he makes a decision regarding treatment and helps him get prepared. I think that when it comes to prostate cancer and sexual function, being surprised is not advantageous. I believe that it is never too early to get this information. I know that soon after prostate cancer diagnosis, men are preoccupied, confused, or even overwhelmed by the need to decide on the preferred treatment. I know it is not an easy task. If someone is at this point, sexual function may not be very high on his list. However, most men are cured of their prostate cancer and long after being cured, the main burden may be recovering their sex life, rather than cancer concerns. Generally speaking, the earlier one does something about his sexual function, the better are the results; and I must emphatically state that there is always something that can be done and there are always options for one to improve his sex life. In summary, if sex is important to you, no matter if you are awaiting prostate cancer treatment or you have already been treated, this essay hopefully will address your concerns.

The Anatomic and Physiologic Basis of Normal Sexual Function and of Sexual Dysfunction Following Prostate Cancer Treatments

Normal sexual function is a very complex process that involves several steps that are interlinked. First we need to have the desire to have sex, to be in a state of mind that we are available for sex, or in other words, to be "horny." Loss of sexual drive may be attributable to psychological factors or hormonal imbalance. Any stress, including health concerns, relationship or family issues, financial or work challenges, moves sex down on the priority list. The human body and mind are programmed in such a way that life threats are dealt with first, and sex comes only after these survival issues have been dealt with. Testosterone, the principal male sex hormone, is essential for healthy sexual drive. The next step is being stimulated by a thought, a sight, or direct touch. The nervous system receives the sexual stimuli, the brain processes this information and interprets this information as sexually arousing and initiates the sexual response. The nervous system delivers a message to the penis to initiate the process of erection. Erections are achieved by increasing the blood flow into the penis and occlusion of the blood drainage out of the penis. The blood-filled penis is larger and rigid, ideal properties for penetration. Oral sex and masturbation do not require a rigid penis, but anal penetration is possible only with adequate penile rigidity. With increasing sexual stimulation, a climax is reached and ejaculation of semen occurs. For semen ejaculation we need a forceful contraction of the seminal vesicles that store the semen and unobstructed outflow channels. The urinary bladder outlet is tightly closed during ejaculation, to prevent urine from leaking out and to prevent semen from escaping backwards, into the urinary bladder. This closure sphincter mechanism is composed of a circular muscle at the bladder neck. There is a second muscle sphincter, further down the urethra, but this sphincter has to be left open to allow the semen to be ejaculated. At the time of ejaculation, there is a sensation that is perceived as enjoyable and rewarding. This sensation is the orgasm and is generated by the brain. Right after sexual activity, ejaculation, and orgasm, we are sexually satisfied, we do not feel the urge to have sex and it is extremely difficult to get an erection again. This stage is termed the "refractory period" and is controlled by hormonal factors acting in the brain: Dopamine and adrenalin shorten the refractory period and serotonin lengthens its duration. The duration of the refractory period is highly variable in men and even in the same person at different ages or states.

Understanding this complex mechanism of normal sexual function is the key to understanding the anatomical and functional changes that occur with prostate cancer treatments. In radical prostatectomy, the prostate and the seminal vesicles, which are essential components of the ejaculatory mechanism, are surgically removed. Thus, immediately after surgery, men become unable to ejaculate semen and there is no recovery or surgical procedure that can reconstruct the ejaculation mechanism. While there is no ejaculation of semen after radical prostatectomy, men not infrequently leak urine during orgasm. Urine leakage after surgery happens because the bladder neck sphincter mechanism is deficient and unable to provide tight bladder closure. The most commonly discussed side effect of radical prostatectomy is the change in erection rigidity, termed "erectile dysfunction." The anatomical basis accounting for erectile dysfunction after radical prostatectomy is injury to the erection nerves, which lie on both sides of the prostate. It is impossible to remove the prostate without some manipulation of these delicate nerves. Even gentle handling of the nerves by an experienced surgeon to tease them away and allow removal of the prostate, may cause temporary or permanent decline in erectile rigidity. Unfortunately, nerve fibers, unlike other tissues in the human body, are extremely slow to heal and recover, accounting for the slow, gradual recovery of erections after radical prostatectomy, a process that may last for many months. It has been suggested that although the main problem causing erectile dysfunction after radical prostatectomy is erection nerves injury, injury to blood vessels during surgery and interruption of normal blood flow to the penis may also contribute to the difficulties men experience trying to achieve erections after surgery.

Radiation (radiotherapy) for prostate cancer also may cause injury to anatomic structures that are essential to sexual function; however, the pattern of injury and the resultant change in sexual performance are very distinct from radical prostatectomy. Initially, during the treatment itself, there are hardly any noticeable changes in the structure or the function of the organs and tissues involved in sexual activity. During and shortly after treatment, men may experience stress, depression, or fatigue, possibly leading to reduced sexual activity that is psychologically based. The impact of radiation on sexual function as well as on prostate cancer cells is a slow, ongoing process. The main mechanism of injury is damage to blood vessels and impairment of penile blood supply. Without the ability to significantly increase penile blood flow, erection cannot be achieved. It has been suggested that the erection nerves may also be adversely affected by radiation, and erectile dysfunction after radiotherapy, therefore, may be a result of damage to both blood vessels and nerves. Unfortunately, unlike after radical prostatectomy, recovery of blood vessels or nerves after radiation has not been described. Even with advances in radiation technology that provide accurate delivery of high dose radiation to the prostate while minimizing the scattered radiation to the neighboring structures, erectile dysfunction may not be avoidable. Similarly, ejaculation is also affected by radiotherapy; most of the semen fluid is normally produced by the prostate and the seminal vesicles. This fluid is transported through delicate channels within the prostate. Radiation to the prostate and seminal vesicles causes gradual cessation of seminal fluid production and obstruction of semen flow due to scarring of the semen channels, and eventually to loss of ejaculation. Sexual drive and orgasm are not commonly affected by radiation and urine leakage during orgasm does not occur.

Hormonal medications are aimed at reducing the principal male hormone, testosterone, to negligible levels, similar to the effect of castration. Testosterone is required for prostate cancer cells growth, and testosterone deprivation is used delay the spread of prostate cancer in men who were not cured by surgery or radiation, or in conjunction with radiation to enhance its effect. However, testosterone deprivation is not without sexual function side effects: Lack of testosterone causes the disappearance of sexual drive and men rarely even think about sex. Very low levels of testosterone are also associated with erectile dysfunction and reduction in semen production. With prolonged testosterone deficiency, lasting more than several weeks or months, the penis undergoes atrophy and degeneration, and permanent erectile dysfunction and reduction in penile dimensions will ensue. Too often the sexual side effects are underestimated or not discussed sufficiently; thus it is important to discuss with one's doctor the oncological benefit of hormone therapy vs. its sexual side effect.

Not infrequently, hormonal treatments are given following other prostate cancer treatments or in combination with radiotherapy. Other possible scenarios of treatment combinations are radiation after radical prostatectomy failure or radical prostatectomy after radiation therapy. In these complex cases of multi-modality management, the injury is synergistic rather than additive: For example, if radical prostatectomy is performed after radiation therapy failure, the expected nerve injury in surgery is greater than the injury in case of radical prostatectomy alone, as radiation effects make preservation of the erection nerves very difficult, even in the hands of expert surgeons.

Radical Prostatectomy and Sexual Dysfunction

All prostate cancer treatments take their toll in many ways when it comes to sexual function. The anatomic and functional basis for the sexual function alterations has been detailed previously. Knowing the sexual function consequences of each treatment, when to expect these changes to appear and whether they are temporary or permanent, will allow one to better understand the expected changes in one's sex life, to get oneself prepared and to minimize the burden associated with adverse sexual consequences of prostate cancer treatments.

Surgery to remove the prostate and the seminal vesicles (radical prostatectomy) is the commonly selected treatment for young, healthy men with localized cancer that has not spread beyond the prostate. The most abrupt change after surgery is the loss of the ability to ejaculate, termed "anejaculation." Men may still have a healthy sex drive, can be sexually aroused, may have erections, enjoy sexual stimulation, and reach satisfactory climax (orgasm). However, during climax, semen will never come out. This is a normal outcome of radical prostatectomy and not a complication. Anejaculation has important implications; men and their partners often derive significant sexual satisfaction from the ejaculation itself. Being unable to ejaculate may be associated with loss of self-esteem and sense of manhood. Moreover, if future fathering of a child from one's own sperm is desired or even considered, it is important to know that it will never be possible to collect sperm naturally for insemination, in-vitro fertilization, or other reproduction procedures after having had a prostatectomy. Discussing sperm banking with one's surgeon before surgery is imperative in order to facilitate future fertility treatments. After radical prostatectomy, sperm can still be extracted directly from the testes, but that requires a surgical procedure.

Although semen ejaculation after radical prostatectomy does not occur, some fluid may come out of the penis, but it is not semen. If it is a thick, whitish fluid in small amount, it is a secretion of urethral glands. These glands are situated along the urine pipe (urethra) and their role is to lubricate the way for the semen. After radical prostatectomy, these glands continue to secrete their fluid, not "knowing" that there is no semen coming anymore. If it is a watery, thin fluid, in different amounts each time, it may be urine. The medical term for ejaculation of urine is "climacturia." It occurs in 20-45% of men after radical prostatectomy and the amount of ejaculated urine varies from a few drops to a lot. Climacturia is more common during the first year after radical prostatectomy. Urine leakage may also occur during sexual activity, before climax. There are several things you should know about urine: urine is sterile and you cannot infect your partner when you ejaculate urine. HIV transmission has not been associated with urine contact. Although you do not ejaculate after radical prostatectomy, you can still get or transmit urethral infection (medically termed: "urethritis"), commonly called Gonorrhea or Chlamydia after the germs that cause this type of infection. Men after radical prostatectomy commonly experience erectile dysfunction hindering penetrative sex; hence oral sex is commonly practiced. Urethritis is commonly transmitted in oral sex and this does not change after radical prostatectomy. You may also wish to make your partner aware of possible urine leakage before he performs oral sex on you. Some drugs, like methamphetamine (referred to as crystal or Tina in the vernacular), are secreted in the urine in significant amounts and their effect on the partner if urine is swallowed depends on the type of the drug, its concentration in the urine, and the amount of urine swallowed by the partner. Ejaculation of urine during sex and orgasm can be minimized or even prevented by emptying your bladder before sexual activity or by using a tight constriction ring (cock ring). After a few attempts you will find the right tightness for you, when it is not too uncomfortable, yet urine does not leak. When using a tight ring, metal rings should be avoided to prevent accidental entrapment of the penis and severe penile damage.

All men experience a certain amount of deterioration in their erection quality after radical prostatectomy. The change in erection rigidity in commonly noticed immediately after surgery, usually after the catheter is removed and men start trying to stimulate themselves and get an erection for the first time after surgery. Some men have partial erections shortly after surgery, others have none. Men who have erection shortly after surgery may experience further deterioration. The low point of erectile function is usually reached at three months after surgery. If the nerves have been well preserved by an experienced surgeon, a recovery of the nerves and erectile function is anticipated. Unfortunately, the recovery process is long and may take eighteen to twenty months or even longer.

Younger age, consistent and sturdy erections before surgery, lack of concomitant significant medical conditions, and well-performed nerve-sparing surgery are all associated with higher chances of erectile function recovery. The current medical literature does not report on any advantage of robotic or laparoscopic surgery over open surgery regarding erectile function recovery. A survey of the highest quality medical publications on erectile function after radical prostatectomy showed that, overall, approximately 60% of men recover their erectile function. This information must be interpreted with great care because in most of these medical publications, recovery is defined as being able to perform vaginal penetration with or without the use of erectile dysfunction pills like Viagra, Cialis, or Levitra. Gay men who wish to regain their ability to have penetrative anal intercourse usually need greater rigidity to penetrate comfortably without struggling. Most men are not able to achieve the desired rigidity right after surgery without using medication. It is advisable to use one of these pills when trying to get erections the first few times after surgery. It is also a good idea to do the first few trials via self-stimulation (masturbation) rather than in a sexual encounter, which may be stressful, especially with an unfamiliar or unsupportive partner or with multiple partners. After the first few experiences, you will know your body better and you will know what to expect. Being surprised with unexpected difficulties in getting an erection in a sexual encounter is not a good idea. As a rule, avoid negative experiences as much as possible. When sex becomes a negative experience, we tend to avoid it and, as time goes by, we give up.

If getting an erection is important to you and pills are not helpful, there are other treatment options. Though Viagra, Cialis, or Levitra are considered magical pills, in the first few months after radical prostatectomy the chances that one will have a decent erection with a pill are only about 25%. Most men use penile injections, at least temporarily while waiting for their nerves to recover. Penile injections are more effective than pills, and the response rate is 80-90%. With penile injections, men inject their penis with a medication that dilates blood vessels and enhances blood flow to the penis. It is important to find a urologist who can teach you how to do it safely, adjust the dose carefully, and prescribe the medication responsibly. While prolonged erections are extremely rare with the use of pills, they can definitely occur with a penile injection overdose. Prolonged erection lasting more than four hours may cause irreversible penile erectile tissue damage if not promptly treated and terminated. If penile injections are not effective, there are still more options to help get erections, such as vacuum devices that pump blood into the penis and induce erection artificially. The blood is kept inside the penis by applying a constriction ring at the base of the penis. Men commonly are unhappy with the vacuum erection devices because the erection does not look or feel normal. If one decides to try the vacuum device, it is imperative to get an FDA-approved product that has a pressure pop-off protection mechanism and not devices sold in sex toy stores. Excessive negative vacuum pressure may cause permanent damage to your penis.

The best option if penile injections fail to get a satisfactory erection is penile implant surgery (penile pump). The penile implant is composed of two inflatable cylinders that are inserted into the penis, a pump that is inserted into the scrotum, and a reservoir of fluid. The implant is inserted surgically and, after recovery, will enable one to get a fully-rigid erection within seconds by pumping up the device; and one can keep an erection as long as he likes. It is important to get detailed information on the pros and cons of penile implant surgery, as this erectile dysfunction treatment is not reversible. Penile implant surgery has very high satisfaction rates. However, it is important to understand that while the penile implant allows one to get full penile rigidity, there is no direct effect on sexual drive, orgasm intensity, or increase in penile length. Men may have secondary improvement in their sexual interest when sex that became a struggle after radical prostatectomy turns to be a positive and enjoyable experience again.

Alterations in the nature of orgasm have also been reported after radical prostatectomy. It is important to understand that orgasm occurs in our brain, not in our penis. Although orgasm usually occurs after intense stimulation of the penis, while the penis is fully erect and during ejaculation, after radical prostatectomy things change. Even if one is unable to get an erection, he can still stimulate himself by masturbation and reach enjoyable orgasm. Changes in the nature of orgasm after radical prostatectomy have not been extensively studied, but a study from Cornell University in New York addressing changes in the nature of orgasm after radical prostatectomy reported that 22% have no change in orgasm, 37% had complete absence of orgasm, 37% had decreased orgasm intensity, and 4% had a more intense orgasm. About one-half of men report pain during orgasm. It is unclear if the changes in orgasm are psychologically based, secondary to the loss of sensations associated with semen propulsion and ejaculation sensation, or attributable to yet to be discovered factors. It is also unknown whether "gay orgasm" is any different from "straight orgasm" and whether these data are applicable to gay men. Changes in the nature of orgasm tend to improve with time; however, it is unknown if it is a process of recovery or adaptation to the new orgasmic pattern. Although it has been suggested that radical prostatectomy may change the anatomy and the innervation of the anal canal, currently there are no studies depicting the changes in the nature of anal sensation, pleasure from sex, or orgasm intensity in gay men who engage in receptive anal sex.

Although penile length, girth, and shape are important to every man's self-esteem and body image, only in the past decade have changes in penile dimensions and shape after radical prostatectomy been described and brought to the attention of surgeons, sexual medicine experts, and patients. Initially, it had been suggested that penile shortening occurs because the surgeon pulls the urethra and the penis to reattach it to the bladder and restore the urinary tract continuity after the prostate is removed and a gap is created. Although this explanation may sound appealing, this is not the case. The urethra and the penis are fixed in place and the bladder is brought down to the urethra, rather than the opposite. Penile shortening happens initially because the nerves that promote erection do not work and the penis is depleted of blood. If blood flow to the penis is restored, the penis will grow to its original length. But if nothing is done to maintain the blood flow, to deliver more oxygen, and to stretch the penis, after several months, the penis undergoes irreversible atrophy and degeneration, it loses its elasticity, and the expansible erectile tissue is replaced by scar tissue. At this point, the penile length and girth changes become permanent. Men who had radical prostatectomy are reported to also have a higher incidence of developing penile deformities. This medical condition, called Peyronie's Disease, was first described in 1743; however, we still don't know its exact cause or mechanism (De la Peyronie, 1743). Peyronie's Disease manifestations include development of penile curvature, narrowing, shortening, and indentations of the penis. These disease deformities are evident only during erection; hence, most men notice them only after being successfully treated for their erectile dysfunction. The association of the disease and radical prostatectomy is poorly understood, but increased risk of this condition has been reported in men who had radical prostatectomy. An interesting study from Memorial Sloan-Kettering in New York showed that gay men with Peyronie's Disease tend to present for medical evaluation earlier than straight men.

Radiation Therapy and Sexual Dysfunction

Erectile dysfunction also occurs after radiation therapy for prostate cancer. A question I am frequently asked is whether a specific type of treatment is associated with higher or lower incidence of erectile dysfunction: radiation compared to surgery, open surgery compared with robotic surgery, or external radiation compared to brachytherapy (seed implant therapy). The answer to this question is not simple. There are no direct high-quality comparative studies that can adequately answer this question. From the current medical literature, it appears that the incidence of erectile dysfunction is similar with all treatment modalities. It must also be remembered that the available data come mainly from centers of excellence and that surgeons and also radiation oncologists differ in their skills, techniques, and obviously in their outcomes. Erectile dysfunction after radiation therapy is first noticed several months or a year after treatment. Over the next year or two, it slowly progresses and then it tends to reach a plateau and stabilize around three years after treatment has been completed. As for radical prostatectomy, good erections before radiation therapy, good general health, and younger age are all associated with better erectile function after treatment. Unlike radical prostatectomy, after which there is sharp decline in erectile function followed by improvement and recovery, the radiation effect on the penis and other structures involved in the erection process is permanent: Once the deterioration in erectile function is evident, recovery does not occur.

Radiation therapy has an effect on ejaculation as well. If the treatment includes radiation delivered from the outside only (external beam radiotherapy), initially there is minimal change, but men do have progressive decline in the amount of ejaculated semen and eventually, the vast majority become unable to ejaculate. With seed implantation (brachytherapy), the decline in ejaculated semen amount may be prompt. Radiation therapy may also cause sperm DNA defects; hence, if future fatherhood is desired, the best strategy is to bank sperm before any treatment.

Peyronie's Disease and penile length alteration occurrence after radiation therapy have never been adequately studied. Currently, there is only one small study showing significant penile shortening after the combined treatment of hormonal medication and external radiation. Unfortunately, there is presently not enough medical knowledge to tell how much penile length you may lose, based on the specific radiation protocol you are about to be treated with. There are also no studies to directly link or refute the occurrence of penile length and girth changes or the development of other penile morphologic changes after radiation therapy. If one is facing a decision regarding prostate cancer treatment, it is advisable to keep up to date with the medical information regarding research progress in this area, including the risk, prevention strategies, and treatment. The patient already treated who notices changes in the shape or the size of his penis may want to seek medical evaluation and information on the available treatment options.

The prostate lies in close proximity to the rectum. All forms of radiation to treat prostate cancer, even when best targeted, deliver some radiation to the rectum. Radiation may cause rectal side effects that one should be aware of, particularly if he is practicing receptive anal sex. We tend to classify rectal side effects as acute side effects, which resolved within six months after radiation therapy completion, and chronic side effects, which continue for more than six months after radiation therapy. Acute side effects may include diarrhea, rectal bleeding, abdominal pain, mucus discharge, and uncommonly, constipation. Chronic rectal side effects may appear late, even two years after treatment, and include urgency (inability to hold the feces and delay defecation), fecal incontinence, rectal pain, rectal stricture, mucus discharge, rectal bleeding, and predisposition to rectal injury and rectal perforation. The reported incidence of rectal side effects varies with different radiation therapy modalities and different doses. In most medical publications, rectal side effects that are more than mild and self-limiting occur in less than 10% of men; however, one should consult his radiation oncologist for information on side effects of the specific radiation protocol prescribed. Needless to say, the radiation oncologist is very unlikely to initiate discussion on rectal sexual dysfunction among gay men. Nor does the medical literature address this question either. However, one needs to be aware of these possible side effects of radiation therapy, as they are not without consequences. Even mild and self-limiting rectal side effects may be bothersome and even worrisome if not expected. Rectal pain may make anal penetration extremely uncomfortable or even impossible; rectal bleeding may increase the risk of blood-borne viral infections such as HIV and Hepatitis C; diarrhea, fecal incontinence and mucus discharge may cause embarrassment and discomfort to both sex partners, and the list goes on. Rectal injury is a life-threatening complication that one needs to be aware of, especially if rectal-insertion of sex toys or "fisting" are among one's sex practices. The irradiated rectum loses it elasticity and becomes extremely vulnerable to injury. This vulnerability is a result of both acute and chronic changes that are induced by the radiation. While the acute changes resolve, the chronic injury remains for a lifetime. Unlike other side effects that are easily noticeable, rectal fragility is noticed only after injury occurs, when it is already too late.

Hormonal Treatment and Sexual Dysfunction

Charles Huggins and C.V. Hodges were the first to discover the association of prostate cancer and testosterone, for which they received the Nobel Prize in physiology and medicine in 1966. They showed that reduction of testosterone levels is beneficial in controlling disseminated prostate cancer. If you are currently taking testosterone or wish to start taking testosterone and you were recently diagnosed with prostate cancer or you were successfully treated for prostate cancer, or if you have disseminated disease, you need to let your doctor know that and discuss the risks and benefits of testosterone supplementation. Traditionally, testosterone was not recommended for men with prostate cancer; however, recent research support the safety of restoring testosterone to normal levels in men who have low testosterone and were successfully treated for prostate cancer. There are no studies regarding the consequences of excessive testosterone levels in prostate cancer survivors. Some men with prostate cancer need testosterone ablation, temporal or permanent, either as additional treatment to radiation therapy or as a sole treatment to control metastatic disease. The first prompt effect of testosterone suppression is loss of sexual drive (libido). Men with low testosterone don't think about sex, even when exposed to sexual content. When they have sex, however, they enjoy it. If you are sexually active in a relationship and you wish to preserve your routine, you need to discuss the loss of libido with your partner. He needs to know that you are very unlikely to initiate sex, but if he initiates sexual activity you will enjoy it. Some men put it on their schedule when they realize that their brain and body cannot spontaneously switch to a state of being "horny." Another issue with hormonal treatment is the loss of ejaculation and sperm production. The consequences of the loss of ejaculation were detailed earlier in this essay, in the discussion of the consequences of radical prostatectomy. However, unlike with radical prostatectomy, where sperm extraction directly from the testes to allow fertility is still possible, hormonal treatment abolishes sperm production and recovery may take many months or even years. Sperm should be banked before hormonal treatment if fatherhood is desired.

Testosterone suppression also has a profound effect on erectile function. While mild decrease in testosterone levels, as commonly seen in older men, does not play a pivotal causative role in the development of erectile dysfunction, when very low levels of testosterone are reached, as with prostate cancer hormonal treatment, erectile function is compromised. After a protracted period, probably several months, of low testosterone, erectile dysfunction becomes permanent, and persists even after testosterone production recovers and normal level is restored. Recovering erectile function after testosterone deprivation therapy, similar to recovery after other treatments, depends on multiple factors such as age, concurrent medical conditions, erectile function before treatment, testicular size and function, and other factors.

Hormonal treatment for prostate cancer also causes changes in penile dimensions. With prolonged testosterone suppression, the penile erectile tissue undergoes degeneration and is replaced by scar tissue as earlier explained in this essay. This structural penile change causes penile shrinkage and shortening as well as loss of girth. A recent study from Harvard Medical School suggests an association between low testosterone and the development of Peyronie's Disease (penile curvature).

Consequences of Treatment Combinations on Sexual Dysfunction

Some men need more than one treatment to cure or to control their prostate cancer. A possible scenario is a man who was treated with radical prostatectomy and recovered well. Several years after his surgery, his PSA starts to rise and he undergoes radiation therapy combined with hormonal treatment. In this case, the erectile mechanism that has recovered from the effects of surgery is not as robust and resilient as in untreated men; therefore the consequences of the additional treatment are more profound. The medical literature suggests that sexual function outcomes of prostate cancer treatments are consistently poorer when initial treatment is compared to a second-line treatment. When discussing sexual side effects of the planned treatment with one's doctor, it is not only important to inform the physician about previous treatments for prostate cancer, but also about the sexual function outcomes of the initial treatment. As a general rule, the better one's recovery from the first treatment was, the better the expected recovery from additional treatments.

Interventions to Prevent and Treat Sexual Dysfunction Following Prostate Cancer Treatments

Most of our understanding and medical knowledge of erectile dysfunction after prostate cancer treatments comes from laboratory and clinical research on men who had a radical prostatectomy; however, the same principals apply to men who had other prostate cancer treatments. Radical prostatectomy was first developed in 1904 at the Johns Hopkins Hospital by Dr. Hugh Young. After surgery, all men lost any ability to achieve erections, since the erection nerves were cut and removed with the prostate. It wasn't until April 26, 1982, that Dr. Patrick Walsh from Johns Hopkins Hospital performed the first nerve-sparing radical prostatectomy and a year later the patient recovered his erections. In the 1980s, the spotlight was on improving the surgical technique allowing for improved nerve-sparing and better erectile function recovery without compromising cancer cure odds. In the 1990s, we gained better understanding of the erection process and became aware of the changes in penile structure and function, as earlier explained. The following decade, the 2000s, was the decade of developing interventions to preserve the penile erectile tissue, waiting for the nerves to recover.

Normally, men have three to six erections every night during the REM sleep, even in men who are not sexually active. Although we do not typically get to experience and derive pleasure from these erections, they are essential to preserve erectile tissue health and integrity. During erection, penile blood flow is increased, more oxygen is delivered to the erectile tissue cells, and the penis is stretched to its full length. Right after prostate cancer treatment, most men lose their ability to achieve erections. This precludes them from being able to quickly resume sexual activity and penetrate; this may last from eighteen to twenty-four months. Not having erections on a regular basis also increases the chances of penile shortening and deformation. No matter what treatment you had, if you cannot achieve erections when you are sexually stimulated or if you do not notice morning erections, you need to do something about it and the sooner, the better. It is exactly like taking a break from the gym: Taking a short break is not a big issue, but taking a two-year break makes it very hard to get back on track and even impossible to get back to where you were. It is important to ask one's surgeon when it is safe to attempt getting erections. Usually it is about a week or two after surgery, once the catheter is removed. During and shortly after radiation therapy or hormonal treatment, it is definitely safe to try to get erections at any time. Getting erections after radical prostatectomy or other treatments is not easy. It is suggested that one try the first few times using one of the pills that promote erection, Viagra, Cialis, or Levitra. One should ask his doctor to prescribe them and buy them only from an authorized pharmacy. Do not settle for the fake, cheap pills offered over the Internet. It is your body and your health after all.

It is important to remember that right after radical prostatectomy pills are effective in only 20 to 25% of men. Getting only a partial erection is probably sound for adequate penile blood flow but not for satisfactory anal penetration. If your erections are not satisfactory, there are other treatment options. Frustration is the biggest enemy. Men who do not perform well in sex tend to lose their sexual drive and eventually give up sexual activity. But there is always something that can be done. If pills don't do the job, there is the option of using penile injections. Penile injections work directly on the erectile tissue inside the penis and can help a man get erections, even if the nerves have not recovered yet. If getting a decent erection after surgery is difficult, using penile injections early after surgery or other treatments will keep the erectile tissue in shape and will increase the chances of erectile function recovery. Most men are satisfied with penile injection, given that the desired response is achieved. Some men may find it difficult to integrate penile injections into their sex life; it depends on one's personality, relationship, sex partner or partners, and particular sex practices. For those men who are hesitant about using the injections, discussing it with their doctor and giving it a trial may ease their concerns and initial fears based on mental images and/or preconceived ideas about putting a needle in one's penis. This decision can affect one's future sex life. The bottom line is if one cannot get erections, even early after treatment, it is imperative to see a doctor, preferably a urologist or a sexual medicine specialist.

In recent years there is growing evidence suggesting that taking a low dose of erection-inducing medications like Viagra is protective to erectile tissue. Men are instructed to take this treatment every day, regardless of their sexual activity. This low dose is very unlikely to give you an erection, but this is not the goal. Medical studies demonstrated that men who used this treatment recovered their erectile function better than men who did not. Men should get more details about daily low-dose erection medication from their doctor.

Coping with all these changes in one's sex life is not an easy task. If a man is in a steady relationship, his partner may need to cope with major changes in their shared sex life, too. Although modern medicine has some good options to help a man get back on the sexual track, this might not be enough. Men and couples coping with prostate cancer can get help and support from sex therapy. A sex therapist will help the couple to improve their communication regarding sex issues with their doctor, their partner or partners, and even with oneself. The individual and the couple can learn how to make the necessary modifications to better adjust to a new sex life. A good sex therapist can also help a man to better integrate erectile dysfunction treatments, such as pills and penile injections, into his sex life and make the most of his new sex life.

Prostate Cancer and Sexual Dysfunction Action Plan

Having read this essay to this point, the reader now understands what changes in sex life to expect after prostate cancer treatments, why these changes occur, and what treatments are available to deal with these changes. What follows is a step-by-step action plan to integrate all this information into a road map that will guide the way toward quickly returning to a satisfying sex life.

1. Relax. Having prostate cancer does not mean, "My sex life is over."

2. Define your information needs. Would you like to get information before you act? Are you often overwhelmed by new information? Do you prefer to get your information in certain ways? Online? Friends? From other people that went through the same experience?

3. Make sure the information you get not only meets your needs, but is also reliable, accurate, and unbiased. For example, the Internet is a great information source, but some websites are trying to sell you something or have an incentive to convince you to make certain decisions.

4. Define your current sex life. What sexual practices do you prefer? Who are your sex partners? Are they a part of your "coping with prostate cancer" journey?

5. Go over all of your treatment options. Rank them by the chances of curing cancer, as well as by the predicted effect on your sex life. Which sex practices can you keep? Which practices will be different and how?

6. Always get the best surgeon or the best oncologist that you can possibly get. Less than optimal treatment given by an inexperienced physician may reduce your chances of cure but also may cause significant side effects, including damaging your sexual function in a way that no sexual medicine expert can ever fix.

7. With issues regarding your cancer care, consult your cancer surgeon or your oncologist. With issues regarding sexual health care, you need to consult a sexual medicine specialist. Cancer surgeons and oncologists tend to focus on the cancer, not on your sex life.

8. When you discuss sexual health issues with professionals, you should tell them about your sexual orientation and your preferred sex practices. Sexual dysfunction management should be tailored to you, rather than "one size fits all."

9. When you discuss sexual health issues with partners, friends, or with prostate cancer survivors, remember that although the information they provide may be valuable, their perspective may be different from yours.

10. Consider every treatment carefully. What is the goal—cure or pain management? What are the chances of success? What are the expected benefits and side effects, including sexual side effects? Once the treatment has been given, there is no way back.

11. Do not delay treatment for sexual health issues. The longer you wait, the fewer your treatment options are and the less satisfactory the results. Too many men wait for their wounds to heal, their PSA to be zero again and again, and their urine continence to be perfect; by the time they decide to take care of their sex life, the damage may have become profound.

12. Saying that, there is always something that can be done to improve your sexual function and to resume pleasurable sex life.

The impact of prostate cancer and its treatment on one's sex life depends on many factors that are related to the individual, his sex practices, his sex partner or partners, his cancer type and extent, his cancer treatments, and other aspects of his life. The first step is to define one's current status and goals. Below are many questions to consider, but there are probably other issues that are important that may not be listed.

Key Questions to Consider Regarding Sexual Function Outcomes Following Prostate Cancer Treatment

Who are you?

1. How old are you?
2. Are you in good health or do you have chronic medical condition?
3. What medication do you routinely take? Do you take testosterone?
4. How do you cope with difficulties and challenges?
5. Do you have a good support system? Friends? Family? Support groups? Health care professionals?
6. What are your expectations?

What are your prostate cancer characteristics?

1. If you have just been diagnosed, what is your PSA level? What are your biopsy results?
2. Do you have localized disease or has the cancer spread beyond the prostate?
3. Is it the first time you are facing prostate cancer or is it a recurrence of a previously treated prostate cancer?
4. What are your prostate cancer treatment options?

Who are your sex partners?

1. Do you have a single partner or multiple partners?
2. If you have multiple partners, are they familiar or usually new? Anonymous?
3. Are your partners or partner the same age you are? Usually younger? Usually older?
4. Are you open about your health status with your partner or partners?
5. Do you think that your partner or partners would be supportive?

What are your sex practices?

1. Are you a very sexual person by nature?
2. Is penetration important to you?
3. Is oral sex important to you?
4. Is ejaculation of semen important to you?
5. Do you use amyl nitrite ("poppers") during sexual activity?
6. Do you use recreational drugs that can adversely affect your sexual function?
7. Do you use medications to help you getting better erections? Do you use other medication or supplements to enhance your sexual performance?

What are the expected sex life changes after your treatment?

1. Do you know when the changes in your sex life are expected to appear?
2. Do you know which changes are temporary and which are permanent?
3. If temporary, do you know how long your sexual function changes are expected to last?
4. Will you have changes in the quality of your erection?
5. Will you be able to ejaculate semen after treatment?
6. Will you have a change in the nature of your orgasm?
7. Is your sexual drive (libido) expected to drop?
8. Are you at risk of changes in your penile dimensions or developing a penile curvature (Peyronie's Disease)?
9. Should you expect further decline in your sexual function, stabilization, or recovery and improvement?
10. Is a future fatherhood of a baby from your own sperm possibly desired?

What are the treatment options to improve your sexual function with prostate cancer?

1. Is there anything you can do before you start prostate cancer treatment?
2. Is the anything you should do during treatment to minimize the adverse effects of sexual-function if your treatment is going to last for a while?
3. Is there anything you should do to enhance your sexual function recovery after treatment?
4. Is there anything you can do to get better erections while waiting for your nerves to recover after surgery?
5. If you desire future fatherhood, what options are available to achieve that goal before and after treatment?
6. What can you do if erection-promoting pills like Viagra, Cialis, or Levitra don't work?

How can you adjust to your new sex life?

1. What are the sexual-function changes that cannot recover?
2. How can you better cope with the changes in your sex life?
3. How can you learn to accept your new sex life?
4. How can you better integrate sexual function therapies into your sex life?
5. How can you educate yourself and your partner or partners about your new sex life?

Conclusion

Prostate cancer and its treatments may cause various forms of sexual dysfunction, including erectile dysfunction, loss of sexual drive, loss of the ability to ejaculate, urine ejaculation during sexual activity or during orgasm, difficulties with receptive anal intercourse, changes in penile length and girth, and possibly even penile curvature (Peyronie's Disease). Sexual dysfunction affects not only men with prostate cancer but also their partner or partners. Knowing the expected changes in one's sex life following prostate cancer treatments allows better treatment selection, better adjustment to these sex life changes, and better coping. Currently, there are interventions that ameliorate the impact of prostate cancer on sexual function and medical research continues to seek ways to improve sexual performance in men with prostate cancer. As a rule, getting the needed information before treatment, selecting the treatment that suits one best, and starting to do something to get back to active sex life will improve a man's chances of sexual function recovery.

Gay Sex after Treatment for Prostate Cancer

Stephen E. Goldstone, MD, FACS and Raanan Tal, MD

Of course being diagnosed with prostate cancer has changed your life and your sex life, but there is life after or with prostate cancer. In this essay, we will give you all the information you need to come to the conclusion that there is also sex life after or with prostate cancer. Yes, you need to educate yourself, your partner if you have one, and the people close to you. It may take some time. However, in this essay, we will give you the tools to overcome the obstacles standing in your way on your journey to your new sex life.

"You've got prostate cancer." These are terrifying words that when first uttered makes it impossible to focus on anything else. Anxiety floods you, maybe you feel like running from the room as the floor slips away beneath you. If you are lucky enough to have a partner or loved one by your side, you squeeze his or her hand to keep your world from ending. You want to live; that is the plain and simple truth, and you will do whatever it takes to beat this disease. Most often the doctor will talk about "treatment options" and you focus on the big picture of what will give you the best chance for survival. You probably won't think about sex because there are too many other things on your mind. Your partner might think about sex, but he won't voice his concerns, fearing that he will sound too petty or too self-involved when your life is at stake. Hopefully your doctor will discuss sex, but he might couch everything in medical terminology, making it difficult to understand. And besides, you rarely hear anything else that is said after the word "cancer."

And then your treatment ends and you lie in bed thankful that you got through it. Maybe a hand reaches under the sheets for you or the usual quick kiss goodnight lingers. Your heart skips beats once again, your breathing quickens, not from sexual excitement but from something else: sexual terror. Sex after treatment for prostate cancer might be the scariest thing you'll have to face after the diagnosis itself.

"Will I be able to have sex again?" is not an easy question for a physician to answer because it depends on a multitude of factors. Hopefully, your doctor will have raised the issue before you underwent treatment, even if you didn't raise it. But still, discussing sex with your doctor early on may not offer much solace when trying to "get it up" that first time. Before discussing sexual function further, we would like to lay out some simple, basic facts that we can identify that help predict sexual function after surgery.

1. The older you are at the time you begin treatment for prostate cancer, the greater the chance that you will have problems with sexual function.

2. If you didn't have problems with sexual function before treatment, you are less likely to have problems after.

3. The more advanced your cancer, the more intensive the treatment is likely to be and therefore the greater the chance that you will experience sexual dysfunction.

4. If your doctor advises Lupron (leurprolide acetate: used for hormonal therapy) to combat the cancer, you will certainly have problems with sexual function. Lupron shuts down the production of your testosterone and will decrease libido and is very likely to cause significant and probably irreversible problems getting erections. The longer you are on Lupron, the greater the likelihood you will experience sexual function problems. Recovery depends on age, health

condition, testicular size and consistency, pre-treatment testosterone production, and so on. There is no cut-off point. If you are young and in great shape you can be on Lupron for a year and recover reasonably well. If you are older and starting from a lower point, a single shot can have a detrimental effect. There is no "cookbook" here, so it is necessary to tailor the discussion about hormone treatment to each patient specifically.

5. Having an understanding partner will help in preserving or restoring sexual function.

Treatment for prostate cancer affects sexual function for two important reasons: The prostate contributes the bulk of the fluid that makes up your semen, and the nerves that stimulate your penis into an erection also run close by. They can be affected by cancer treatment. In addition, anal sex, which may be an integral part of a gay man's sex life, can also be affected by treatment for prostate cancer. Sexual function can depend greatly on whether or not your treatment was surgery or radiation therapy. It is best to discuss the various issues specific to each treatment.

Radical Prostatectomy

Surgical treatment for prostate cancer is called a "radical prostatectomy." As has been discussed elsewhere in this book, the surgery removes the entire prostate gland and some surrounding tissue. The doctors try to spare the nerves that stimulate your erection, but sometimes nerve injury cannot be avoided as the surgeon tries to cure your cancer. The larger and the more aggressive your tumor is, the less likely it is that your surgeon can spare your erection nerves without compromising the chance for your cure of cancer. Most, if not all, men will notice significant change in erections, even after what is called "nerve-sparing" surgery. As one urologist likes to put it, "It is more like a 'soft on' rather than a 'hard on'. It is also common to have initial problems with erections (you may not be able to get one at all right after surgery) that do improve with time. It can take as long as two years for your erections to stabilize. The important thing is not to get discouraged and to discuss these problems with your doctor.

The other universal phenomenon after radical prostatectomy surgery is an inability to ejaculate. As we have previously said, most of the semen is produced by the prostate and seminal vesicles. The sperm cells are produced by the testicles, however they comprise only about 2% of you ejaculate. When the surgeon removes your prostate and your seminal vesicles and disconnects the vas deference on both sides (the pipes that carry the sperm cells from your testicles to the prostate), there is no production of the seminal fluid and therefore nothing comes out during orgasm. This is a situation that is very different from prostate surgery for benign, non-cancerous disease. In surgery for a benign enlarged prostate called a benign prostate hyperplasia (BPH), the prostate and the seminal vesicles are left in place; the vas is also left intact but the muscle that closes your bladder so your ejaculate moves out of your penis, rather than back into your bladder, is destroyed. Instead your ejaculation becomes retrograde and shoots into your bladder. After surgery for benign disease some men are able to ejaculate, although with reduced amount; after radical prostatectomy, there is no ejaculation. While you still experience the feeling of an orgasm, nothing comes out. This can be a very troubling, albeit normal, result of surgery for both you and your sexual partner. Some men or their partners feel that they aren't really sexually satisfied if nothing comes out. Semen is erotic for many gay men. They like to see it, feel it, and taste it. Inability to ejaculate (called anejaculation) can rob them of this very important stimulant.

Fortunately, radical prostate surgery does not affect

your anus or rectum. Once you get over the pain from surgery and your incision fully heals, you will be able to have anal sex again without restriction. Nor is there any evidence to suggest that anal sex caused your prostate cancer; nor will it cause it to come back.

Radiation Therapy

Radiation can be given either as external beam (the machine is positioned outside your body) or through radioactive seeds implanted directly into your prostate (brachytherapy). Your doctor will advise you which type of treatment is best for your particular case. Like surgery, radiation does affect sexual function in some very important ways.

Radiation works by destroying the cancer cells and to some extent the normal tissue around it. The effects of radiation to the surrounding tissue can increase with time and this is the major difference from surgery. The likelihood is that you will have sexual dysfunction immediately after surgery, but it will hopefully improve with time. Radiation, however, can allow you to have normal erections during and immediately after treatment that can weaken or disappear with time. Gradual onset of erectile dysfunction can begin weeks to years after radiation therapy and the severity can vary from just a softer erection to complete erectile dysfunction. Erection problems typically start six to twelve months after radiation, worsen over the first two to three years after radiation, and then stabilize. But as one radiation oncologist likes to advise, "Use it or lose it." Many doctors agree that if you maintain an active sex life, you are more likely to preserve your ability to get erections after radiation treatments.

As mentioned, radiation also gradually destroys your prostate. This can lead to a diminished amount of ejaculate (semen). You may notice a smaller and smaller "load" shoot out and this can be troubling for the reasons outlined above. Sure, you still have the orgasm, but some men may feel less masculine because so little comes out.

Your ability to have anal sex after radiation therapy can depend on the type of radiation you receive. Newer radiation techniques allow for a more focused delivery of the radiation to your prostate, meaning higher dose aimed at your prostate where your cancer is and lower dose to the surrounding tissues. The more focused the radiation is, the lower the dose the rectum receives and thus less damage is done to your rectum. When radiation does hit your rectum it causes severe irritation, diarrhea, and even rectal bleeding. This can make the rectum sore and anal sex uncomfortable. Fortunately, doctors prescribe medications (steroid enemas and anti-diarrhea drugs) to help combat radiation side effects. After your radiation ends, your symptoms should subside, making anal sex once again possible. Rarely, however, does the rectal irritation persist and you experience bloody diarrhea. If that is the case, anal sex will probably not be possible.

What to Do

Communication with your doctor and your partner, if you have one, is critical. Many times gay men are embarrassed to speak with their physicians about sexual function. If we have been taught that our sexuality is an aberration then we have no justification to discuss it with our doctors—right? WRONG. Even if your doctor is uncomfortable speaking about gay sex (and most will be) you need to bring it up. Your doctor might just surprise you and readily answer your questions without the homophobia that you feared. If you have a partner, then it is always best to bring him along for frank discussions about sexual function for very important reasons. Your partner needs to hear what the doctor says so that he can better understand what you are going through. His presence will also help "break the ice" and let your doctor know that you have a same-sex relationship. If you don't have a partner and list yourself as "unmarried" on the typical medical office patient information form, your doctor may incorrectly assume that you don't have sex. Hopefully as physicians become more enlightened, they will not make this inaccurate assumption and will ask even "unmarried" patients whether or not they have sex and with whom.

Erectile dysfunction, whether it is a weaker erection or no erection at all, can be devastating for obvious reasons. If anal sex was an important part of your sexual relationship, then you need a stronger erection to penetrate a man's anus than you would if you had vaginal sex. To have anal sex you must first pass the sphincter muscles that keep your partner's anus closed. The vagina does not have these muscles. A weaker erection might not get through the anal sphincter muscles. Even if your erection starts out strong, difficulties struggling to enter your partner may cause stress, release of adrenalin, a potent hormone that constricts blood vessels and counteracts erection, and suddenly everything goes limp. Moreover, if you have protected sex, the condom may decrease your sensation, diminish stimulation, and increase your chances of erectile dysfunction. Some men find that while they attain a reasonably good erection initially, it does not last long enough for them to climax. No matter which of these problems you experience, you do have sexual dysfunction and your doctor can help.

The most common treatment for failed or weak erections is medication, a pill. Viagra was the first effective erectile dysfunction treatment, followed by Levitra and Cialis. All these pills have been shown to be effective and safe erectile dysfunction treatments, and are manufactured by reputable and trusted pharmaceutical companies. However, if pills fail, don't get discouraged: There are other medications and treatments that are more effective for men after prostate cancer treatments, as well as the potential for surgery. You need to discuss with your doctor the pros and cons of every treatment, so you have the tools to make a decision regarding the treatment that is right for you. If your erection is strong enough for oral sex but not anal sex and you want to have anal sex, you still have a problem and a reason to ask for help. If your doctor won't listen to your concerns about anal sex, then find another doctor. You have a right to speak frankly with your doctor and to expect your doctor to listen and help.

Although most doctors will not recommend it, a cock ring can help if you have problems maintaining an erection. A cock ring works by tightening around veins at the base of your penis that let blood drain out of your erection. The ring acts like a tourniquet and keeps the blood inside the erectile tissue in your penis. A cock ring needs to be tight enough to keep the blood in place but not so tight that it is uncomfortable or can't be removed. Once you reach orgasm, remove it to allow your erection to naturally subside. We recommend an elastic cock ring or one with Velcro or snaps that can always be undone. Go on line or into a gay-themed sex shop and I am sure the man behind the counter can help you find the cock ring that will work best for you.

Speaking frankly with your partner (whether he is a life partner that you've been with for years or a partner that you met minutes before doesn't matter) is crucial for sexual satisfaction. If you are worried that your erection won't last or be hard enough, then explain this to him. Explain to him why you use a cock ring, why you take Viagra, Levitra, or Cialis, or need to inject something into your penis to get hard. Clearly this is easier to do with someone you have a relationship with and it may seem impossible with a guy you just picked up. Either way, go for it. You might just be surprised by his response. If the guy is worth having sex with, he will hopefully be understanding and help you along. Who knows, you might discover that he has been through prostate cancer himself.

This brings us to another avenue for help: support groups. There are support groups for men who've had prostate cancer and these can be very helpful as you struggle to come to terms with your illness and the complications that arise from treatment. Ask your doctor about groups in your area. Call the local gay community center and inquire about similar gay groups. If none exist, why not think about starting one yourself? I assure you that you won't be the first gay man in your town to have struggled through prostate cancer.

While erectile dysfunction can often be successfully treated, inability to ejaculate or diminished ejaculate is not a problem that can be remedied. And again, this is where communication with your doctor and partner(s) can be vital. You need to understand that you are still a sexually functioning man, even if nothing shoots out of your penis. While this can seem obvious, it often isn't. It's one thing to understand in your head that your manhood doesn't depend on your ejaculation, but it is another thing to understand it in your loins. We watch porn movies where the guy shoots a load that could fill a small pond, and his erection is hard enough to knock down small buildings in his way. And what do you have? A limp noodle and little or no load. It gets worse: The guy in the porno video is a twinky while you're old enough to be his father or, heaven forbid, his grandfather. As gay men, we place too much value on youth and virility, and if you allow yourself to buy into this notion it can drastically affect your ability to have satisfying sex. Therapy and support groups can help both you and your partner come to terms with your new sexual function. Malecare is one such group serving gay men who have been diagnosed and/or treated for prostate cancer.

If you've enjoyed being the receptive partner for anal

sex and suddenly you feel that you can't, then you need to speak with your doctor. For gay men, admitting that they enjoy receptive anal sex can be the hardest discussion they need to have. Talking about receptive anal sex might make you feel less like a man; in your eyes and in your doctor's eyes. Fortunately, radiation injury to the rectum often heals with time and the doctor can prescribe enemas or suppositories. If you still bleed when you attempt anal sex despite all available treatments, then you might not be able to have it. On the other side of the fence, men who have been more used to penetrating might consider experimenting with the pleasures of being receptive.

When you first attempt anal sex, it is important that you use a lot of water-soluble lubricant. Don't use lubricants with nonoxynol-9, as these are even more irritating to the rectum. If you use lubricated condoms, these may or may not contain nonoxynol-9. It seems to get more and more difficult to read the tiny print on condom boxes, so we advise buying non-lubricated condoms. That way you know you're not getting ones with nonoxynol-9; besides, there never is enough lubricant on the condom for anal sex anyway.

No matter how badly you want your partner inside you, the act of him trying to enter you causes your anal sphincter muscles to close involuntarily. If you are sore from prior cancer treatments, it can make the pain worse and your partner could tear the delicate lining of your anus and rectum. Even if you are experienced at receptive anal sex, it might have been some time since you last had it, often before you began cancer treatments. To make it easier on yourself, we advise sitting down on your partner first. That way you control the penetration, and if it hurts you can stay there and wait for the sphincter muscles to relax. It usually takes thirty to sixty seconds before you feel the muscles loosen and then you can sit the rest of the way down on him. While touching your penis may make you more sexually aroused and less focused on the discomfort, it activates a reflex that causes your sphincter muscles to tighten further. After penetration, move up and down on him a few times and then if you want you can switch to whatever position you like. And who knows, you might discover that you like being "on top," so to speak. If you do feel irritation or notice some bleeding, stop and rest for a day or two. When you try again, experiment with other positions to see if that makes a difference. Some positions will put less stress on your rectum than others and might help you have satisfying anal sex.

If you have HIV then it is still necessary to have protected anal sex after prostate cancer. Even if you no longer shoot a full load, or any load for that matter, fluid or reduced ejaculate that comes out can carry HIV and is capable of infecting an HIV-negative partner.

Treatment after prostate cancer can cause your sphincter muscles to tighten if you've had a lot of rectal irritation. The irritation can send your sphincters into spasm, especially if an anal tear (fissure) had developed. Surgery can also predispose you to developing a fissure because the pain medication you needed during healing is constipating. Either diarrhea (from radiation) or hard bowel movements (from constipation) can tear the delicate anal lining. Sphincter muscles in spasm can feel as if they have been working out at a gym. They tighten and build more muscle mass. When you try to have anal sex again, you may feel too tight. If this is the case, I recommend that you buy a small dildo. And we do mean small—about the size of your thumb. You can have an erection while you gently insert the dildo, but don't touch your penis. As previously detailed, touching your penis may cause the anal sphincter muscles to tighten and makes it even harder to get the dildo in. Once it is in, it is safe to masturbate if you desire, and see how it feels. If the dildo becomes pleasurable, then try a little larger one. It might take weeks of gradually increasing the size of the dildo to stretch your anus so that you can accommodate your partner. With time, hopefully you will enjoy anal sex again.

If you find that you simply can't have anal sex or even if you can't maintain an erection, it doesn't mean that all is lost. If your rectum can't be used for sex, don't lose sight of the fact that you still have your mouth and hands and many other body parts. They can still be used to satisfy both you and your partner. If you enjoy penetrating your partner, don't give up yet, even if pills or penile injections to induce erections do not work. The most effective way to get you back on track is having a penile implant (penile prosthesis or penile pump) inserted. It will require surgery, but you will be discharged from hospital the same day or the next morning, and after a short recovery process, you will be able to achieve a fully rigid erection within seconds, whenever you want lasting as long as you want. Of all erectile dysfunction treatments, penile prosthesis surgery has the highest treatment patient satisfaction rate. Of course, before you make your decision whether you are going for the surgery, you need to discuss the risks and benefits with your surgeon. See the essays on penile implants in this volume.

It is impossible to expect that the diagnosis and treatment of prostate cancer won't affect your sex life. Fear of sex is very common. You or your partner might worry that ejaculation can spread the cancer from you to him. It can't. Others worry that sex could cause the prostate cancer to come back. It can't. Sex did not cause your cancer in the first place and it won't cause it to come back. Partners often worry that sex causes pain or that your weaker erection or failure to ejaculate means you're not being satisfied. You must reassure him that what he does gives you pleasure and the fact that you don't shoot like the old days doesn't mean your orgasms aren't as strong as the ones you had before the cancer.

Fear, whether real or imagined, can conspire to keep you and/or your partner from attempting sex. If you've been together for a long time, your desire for each other may not be what it was when you first met. You probably haven't had sex during the treatment and recovery period, which can stretch from weeks to months. It may feel like you've simply "gotten out of the habit" of having sex. But just like the guy who fell off the horse and got right back on, that is what you need to do. You might even go off for a romantic weekend or perhaps put in a porno DVD to crank up the sexual heat. Communicate about your fears and worries, and this will help you both confront the problem. And then do whatever it takes to restore your sex life.

If you and your partner did not have sex before your prostate cancer and treatment, and especially if you were not having sex with anyone, it will be harder to overcome sexual dysfunction. You should try to masturbate. Don't be afraid to use sexual aids like dildos or other toys or to watch porn. Even if you don't obtain an erection, it can still feel good. Go with it and you just might reach an orgasm without ever getting hard. If nothing comes out, then so what? An orgasm is still an orgasm. If something does come out, don't be frightened of a little urine. Sex after prostate cancer will be difficult, and you might need much more stimulation to get going again. Whether you have a partner or do it by yourself, hopefully after the initial difficulty the situation improves as your relax more and fears subside. Just remember that it will never get better unless you try.

For the Partners

We cannot overemphasize the importance of communication. If your loved one has been treated for prostate cancer, chances are that it has affected you as well. Sure, you worried about what he had to endure, offered encouragement to get him through the treatment, and worried that you might lose your life partner to this terrible disease. You were scared but you didn't voice these fears because you needed to keep up the brave façade. And all through it you probably felt very alone. If you have a monogamous relationship, you also haven't had sex during the treatment and recovery period and the need for physical intimacy is probably very frustrating.

Now that the treatment is over, you are probably just as scared about touching him as he is about being touched. Communicate these fears and it will help you both get back on track. It is important that you bring up issues with him and with the doctor. Patients may not talk to their doctors about sexual problems, but then that is where you come in. You can give voice to the issues he is too afraid of or too embarrassed to discuss. We are not telling you to go behind his back (although sometimes that is necessary) but to tell your loved one that you both need to discuss the sexual issues with the doctor at the next office visit. If he says that he can't talk about it, then offer to bring it up for him. You can write out the questions beforehand so he understands exactly what will be asked. That way there are no surprises. Hopefully, as the discussion you initiated unfolds he will join in. It even helps if you notify the doctor's office beforehand. Tell the receptionist that you may need a little extra time to speak about personal matters with the doctor. With luck he or she will build extra time into your appointment so you and the doctor don't feel rushed. It is always wrong to bring up the sensitive issue of sex as an afterthought as the doctor heads toward the exam room door. If you do speak to the doctor alone about problems you and your partner may have, don't be put off if particulars of your partner's condition are avoided. Given privacy regulations, it may be impossible for the doctor to discuss your partner's medical care with you. That doesn't mean that the doctor can't listen to what you've got to say and bring it up at a future visit.

When it actually comes time to initiate sex (and that might be what you have to do), take it slow. Gentle caressing and well-placed kisses can go a long way to quieting fears and letting your partner feel safe in your bed. If his penis fails to rise to the occasion, don't take it as a sign that you are doing something wrong. Your partner can still be aroused even to the point of an orgasm without getting an erection. If you sense that he is frustrated, you might need to back off, offer reassurance, and then begin again. Ask what makes him feel good and be aware of more subtle cues that tell you he's aroused. His erection might be gone, so pay attention to the rhythm of his breathing or soft sounds he may make. Guide his hand to your own penis and show him that you find pleasuring him stimulating, too. Whipping you into a frenzy might be enough to reassure your loved one that he still is desirable.

Last but not least, gay men are not saints. Hurt feelings and fears of inadequacy, undesirability, and even that you aren't a man anymore are not uncommon after treatment for prostate cancer. Just as the doctor provides surgery or radiation therapy to combat the physical aspects of this disease, both you and your partner might also need emotional support. This can come in the form of an understanding lover, a physician not afraid to listen to your fears, a therapist, or a support group. And please don't forget that treating the cancer is not enough; your doctor can also treat some treatment consequences such as erection problems. But doctors are not mind readers and they won't know you've got a problem unless you speak up. Don't be afraid to seek help. Life has thrown you both a difficult curve, but with time and above all love and understanding you will get through this. Life is definitely worth living.

Incontinence and Prostate Cancer

Matthew L. Lemer, MD

Santillo and Lowe, in this volume, provide an excellent overview of how urinary dysfunction affects the quality-of-life issues after prostate cancer treatment. I aim to expand the scope of this discussion and to describe the specific therapies available to manage them. This is for the patient who is about to be treated for prostate cancer or who has already been treated and is grappling with urinary problems, or for the lover, friend, or relative of someone like this. It is intended to empower them.

It does not take long after a patient has completed treatment for prostate cancer to begin to realize the psychological and physical changes. He may be tired, confused, grateful, and depressed. He may find himself involuntarily squirting urine onto the protective continence pad his doctor has instructed him to wear. This squirting may happen when he gets out of bed, walks, or returns to the gym. He may leak urine and not even be aware of when or why it occurred. He may make more frequent trips to the bathroom to urinate. He may wake up at night to urinate now that he has been treated but never had this problem beforehand. He may worry that he might not be able to control the urge to urinate if he hesitates to get up in the middle of a movie or the theater or is stuck in unanticipated traffic. Advances in radiation modalities and surgical techniques continue to reduce the likelihood that a patient will suffer long-term urinary side effects of treatment. But, as I've heard many doctors say, if a patient is one of the small percentages of patients who unfortunately have the problem, his likelihood has now become 100%.

The nature of the urinary problems that may exist depends on the specific method of treatment a patient chooses. As has been already discussed in this book, there are surgical and non-surgical treatments for prostate cancer. Surgical treatments include radical prostatectomy and cryotherapy. Non-surgical treatments include different types of radiation: external beam radiotherapy, radioactive seed implantation (also called brachytherapy), and a combination of modalities. Non-surgical treatments encompass hormonal therapies and "watchful waiting." Hormonal therapies, aimed at decreasing circulating testosterone, do not exacerbate urination. Generally, as the prostate shrinks in response to the hormones, urination actually improves somewhat. "Watchful waiting," or observation without specific intervention, is associated with few urinary problems even after several years.

The main urinary problems that occur after radical prostatectomy are urinary incontinence or leakage, dribbling after urinating, and urinary frequency and urgency. Radiation less commonly can cause incontinence and urgency, too. Men may complain of local burning, particularly after radiation treatments that incorporate radioactive seeds.

Although healthy men generally take urinary control for granted, it requires the coordination of complex processes. Broadly speaking, urinary control involves (1) storage and (2) emptying of urine. Storage of urine requires a stable, elastic bladder and a sufficiently strong, "competent" urinary sphincter and pelvic muscles. In this model, the bladder does not contract while it is filling with urine. It contracts only when a man voluntarily makes the effort to urinate. The urethra, prostate, urethral sphincter (yes, there is another one besides the anal sphincter), and pelvic muscles together constitute the urinary outlet and normally maintain resting tone and resistance to prevent urine from escaping. Even with the typical daily fluctuations of pressure exerted on the bladder from the abdominal muscles, the seal is secure. Emptying of urine requires a strong bladder muscle to expel its contents and a coordinated relaxation of the downstream muscles to minimize outlet resistance.

Stress Urinary Incontinence

The most significant urinary problems after treatment of prostate cancer occur because of a reduction in the body's ability to store urine. By far the most common urinary issue after surgery is stress urinary incontinence, the involuntary loss of urine that generally occurs with activity when the sphincter is weak and cannot compensate for increases in abdominal pressure. Activities that are commonly associated with this form of incontinence are coughing, sneezing, and straining (e.g. moving furniture, picking up a suitcase, defecating, weight-lifting, gardening, getting out of a car, having sex).

The external urethral sphincter, which normally totally prevents stress urinary incontinence in a man, lays immediately adjacent to the prostate and can be easily traumatized or injured with surgical dissection. All men will leave the hospital with a catheter in their penis after surgery for a period of days to weeks. Robotic radical prostatectomy significantly reduces the time the catheter remains in place. Almost all men will experience some stress urinary incontinence in the doctor's office when the catheter is finally removed. This does not mean he is now permanently incontinent. All patients should anticipate this and expect initially that they will need to buy and use absorptive pads.

Urge Urinary Incontinence

The other main form of urinary incontinence after prostate cancer treatment is urinary urge incontinence, a sudden involuntary loss of urine that occurs when the bladder muscle is spastic. Urinary urge incontinence occurs as a complication after radical prostatectomy and radiation therapy. Local tissue irritation and inflammation, altered anatomy, and disruption of neuromuscular pathways can result in bladder spasms even when a man has no intention of urinating. Seemingly, for no reason, a man may be overwhelmed by a strong urge to urinate that results in urine escaping before he can get to the bathroom. It could happen even when the bladder is not full. Patients frequently mention that hearing running water, consuming alcoholic and caffeinated beverages, and changing position from sitting to standing are activities that pronounce this tendency. Most of us have searched for a key to open the door and experienced an intense urge to urinate. Generally, even though we may feel uncomfortable or desperate to get to the bathroom, we will not leak. On the other hand, when a man has involuntary bladder spasms, he more often cannot abort the involuntary bladder muscle contractions and, while he is fidgeting with his house key, will experience urinary urge incontinence. Bladder spasms will also cause increased urinary urgency and frequency in the daytime and nighttime. Urologists refer to urgency, frequency, nocturia (the urge to urinate while sleeping), and urge incontinence as "irritative lower urinary tract symptoms."

Radical Prostatectomy vs. Radiation Therapy

It has been consistently shown that prostate cancer patients treated with radical prostatectomy have higher rates of urinary dysfunction than men treated with external beam radiation. When urinary function was evaluated twenty-four months after treatment for localized prostate cancer, 9.6% of men reported no control or frequently dripping after radical prostatectomy versus 3.5% after radiation therapy; 13.8% reported leaking two or more times per day after surgery versus 2.3% after radiation; 28.1% wore pads to stay dry after surgery versus 2.6% after radiation. There was no difference in urinating frequently between the two groups. When incontinence was defined as needing to wear one or more pad per day to control urinary leakage three years after treatment, 12.3% were incontinent after radical prostatectomy (9.4% nerve-sparing, 15.1% non-nerve-sparing), 2.7% after external beam radiotherapy, 5.4% after low-dose brachytherapy, and 7% after high-dose brachytherapy.

Since prostate cancer patients treated with radical prostatectomy are more likely to develop urinary incontinence, any man considering surgery should understand the likelihood and magnitude of the short-range and long-range urinary outcomes. I see many gay and heterosexual men in my practice who consult me for management of their post-operative urinary problems. Weeks or months have passed since undergoing a radical prostatectomy and they are dismayed that they have not returned to their baseline urinary function. The lack of a quick resolution can be frustrating and disturbing. They may feel less youthful, vibrant, and sexy. They may fear that friends or co-workers have smelled urine on them. And, with leakage, they may be embarrassed to date and have sex. In truth, at least one patient found success through an Internet dating site where he was embraced for his proclivity! It is important to underscore that urine is not considered infectious. While HIV has been found in urine, it is not concentrated in an amount sufficient for transmission.

The fact is that urinary incontinence after a radical

prostatectomy significantly improves over time and can continue improving incrementally even at twenty-four months. At six months, 16.9% of men reported frequent leakage. That figure reduced to 10.9% at twelve months and 6.8% at twenty-four months. At six months, 29% reported having more than two incontinent episodes per day. Only 15.4% of men still had that complaint after twelve months and 11.9% at twenty-four months. Even in the most severe circumstances, where 5.4% reported no control over urination at six months, only 2.8% at twelve months and 1.6% at twenty-four months were still plagued.

In contrast, men with prostate cancer who are treated with external beam radiation have less severe urinary dysfunction initially after treatment and remain that way over time. One published study revealed that after external beam radiation 92% of men had total urinary control and another study showed that 62% had total urinary control. Men who leak after radiation are much more likely to experience urinary urge incontinence (usually associated with a sudden uncontrollable urge with no obvious precipitating event) in contradistinction to those men who leak after radical prostatectomy who are more likely to experience stress incontinence (usually associated with activity that increases intra-abdominal pressure). Men treated with radioactive seed implantation commonly report burning with urination but it is typically mild. In one study, 85% of men experienced burning with urination one month after treatment. 61.5% of them at six months and 66.9% at twelve months had resolution to their pre-treatment baseline level.

Larger body mass index, older age, increased size of prostate, and the presence of preoperative urinary dysfunction and concomitant diseases (e.g. diabetes, hypertension) have all been reported, albeit without complete agreement in the literature, to increase the risk of urinary incontinence after surgical treatment. On the other hand, higher earned income and a married status have been shown to decrease the risk. It can be helpful to use these statistics to counsel patients on treatment choices. Unfortunately, there are no published studies dedicated to looking at urinary dysfunction and prostate cancer treatment in gay men. If being married is associated with a more favorable urinary outcome after treatment, does that also hold true for partnered gay men? We do not have those answers yet.

Quality-of-Life

It is important for one to understand when looking at incontinence rates in this essay or in books that those figures do not necessarily predict satisfaction with treatment or the impact of incontinence on pre-treatment quality-of-life. For example, a man who occasionally leaks urine only during his most physically active times might not be bothered by the leakage. He might have figured out that he can wear a small incontinence pad in his underwear before exercise and not need to worry. Or, in another example, even though he still might use two large pads daily, his gratitude for surviving cancer may far outweigh the displeasure of his incontinence. That man would have a poor score on an incontinence scale but have a much more favorable score on a urinary function quality-of-life scale. Since published incontinence rates alone do not tell the whole story, it is critical to understand Health Related Quality-of-life (HRQoL) statistics.

The field of HRQoL research has exploded recently because it tells a patient what he really wants to know: "When I make the decision to treat my prostate cancer with surgery or with radiation, how distressing will it be after treatment to cope with the inevitable associated side effects?" In other words, "How will my treatment affect my physical, emotional, mental, and social well-being?"

General HRQoL questionnaires ask about physical function (e.g. vigorous activity, lifting, climbing, bending); role limitations due to physical health problems (e.g. accomplishing less, limiting in kind); vitality (e.g. being energetic and full of life); mental health (e.g. depression, nervousness, peacefulness); social functioning (e.g. extent and time in social activity); bodily pain (e.g. magnitude of pain and level of interference) and general health. Disease-specific HRQoL questionnaires assess urinary quality-of-life through questions about function and bother of urinary control, frequency of leaking, wearing of pads, and urinary frequency.

In a study examining HRQoL of urinary function with treatment of prostate cancer, the radical prostatectomy group had worse quality-of-life (QoL) than the external beam radiation group, which, in turn, had worse QoL than the observation only group. With regard to HRQoL of sexual function with treatment, this same pattern was observed. Some studies showed that bowel function HRQoL was worse with external beam radiation than with surgery but other studies showed no difference. Interestingly, there was no difference in general HRQoL among all the treatment groups. The take-home message here is that a man with prostate cancer will have good physical and emotional well-being no matter what treatment decision he makes. Depression, anxiety, alcohol abuse and drug abuse—all prevalent in the gay male population—negatively impacted general HRQoL after treatment.

There are also longitudinal studies where HRQoL is evaluated initially after treatment and at later time points. In one such study, urinary HRQoL declined immediately after surgery but improved at one year; urinary HRQoL was good immediately after radiation and observation and stayed that way at one and two years; sexual HRQoL was poor in all groups and at all time points; general well-being declined initially with surgery and radiation but improved for both by one year. Another study reported their HRQoL findings in a different way. After radical prostatectomy, 61% recovered pre-treatment urinary function by one year; 31% recovered pre-treatment sexual function by one year; 96% recovered pre-treatment bowel function by one year; and 86 to 97% recovered pre-treatment general HRQoL by one year.

It has been shown that husbands and wives often have different preferences regarding treatment when the husband has been diagnosed with prostate cancer. When deciding how to treat his prostate cancer, a man would sacrifice some life expectancy for fewer side effects and a better quality-of-life. She, on the other hand, would want him to live longer even if his life with her is marked by a moderate amount of urinary incontinence and impotence. Unfortunately, there is no information about how male same-sex partners/spouses think about these issues. As gay men with prostate cancer begin to decide how they will treat their disease, it would be useful for them to know what their spouses might be thinking. Are gay spouses generally prone to minimize the importance of urinary and sexual side effects for the sake of improved longevity—like the wives mentioned in the aforementioned study of heterosexual couples—or not.

A frightened man with prostate cancer sitting in his urologist's office would like to think that his doctor is accurately reading his thoughts and needs as he is contemplating his treatment choices. But we know that his urologist is likely to make inaccurate assessments. We, as urologists, tend to emphasize the treatment choice that will confer the greatest chance of cure and life expectancy. We deemphasize quality-of-life considerations, which may be paramount in our patients' minds.

Treatment

Pelvic Muscle Exercises

In my opinion, the most significant thing a patient can do to improve urinary incontinence after prostate cancer treatment is to learn and vigilantly perform pelvic floor muscle exercises, commonly referred to as Kegel exercises. The pubococcygeal muscles, which form a hammock to support the pelvic organs and the urinary sphincter, can be rehabilitated. In my experience, many urologists after surgery casually inform patients that they will do well to perform Kegel exercises. It is usually quickly demonstrated to the patient when the catheter is removed ("squeeze your muscles like you're trying to hold in your urine") or patients are sent home with a pamphlet, which describes the technique in greater detail. This is not the optimal time to learn an important new skill. Patients are overwhelmed with their physical recovery and distracted by fears such as, "Was all my cancer removed?" "I can't believe I need to wear a diaper," "Am I still attractive?" In addition, contrary to general opinion, it is not easy to do Kegel exercises well. Even when patients nod their heads affirming that they know what they are being asked to do, many will incorrectly use their abdominal, gluteal, or leg muscles. Even when they are practicing with the correct muscles, they may be capable of doing them with greater proficiency. I recommend that patients learn and practice the exercises before they have surgery. That way, when their catheter is removed (patients should never do them with the catheter still in place), they can immediately begin in earnest. In my opinion, pelvic floor muscle training with biofeedback is the most superior way to rehabilitate the pelvic muscles. Biofeedback is a way for a patient to learn cues about his body functions that may not be obvious to him. Learning to identify which muscles need to be relaxed to initiate urination and which muscles need to be contracted to stop urination will help the patient minimize involuntary urine leakage. A physical therapist can illustrate this to a patient by externally applying skin electrodes to his pelvic muscles or inserting a finger, weight, or manometer inside his rectum. When the patient contracts his muscles as instructed, he can immediately view from any of these measuring devices how well he is performing the contraction.

It is important to know that Kegel exercises will help reduce both major forms of urinary incontinence after prostate cancer treatment: stress urinary incontinence and urge urinary incontinence. I recommend that patients do the exercise several times per day, ten to fifteen repetitions at a time, ultimately increasing the contraction time to ten seconds. There are also specific opportunities during the day where it is especially helpful to employ the Kegel maneuver. For men predominantly dealing with stress urinary incontinence after a radical prostatectomy, I recommend they contemplate what activities during the day are associated with incontinence and then, seconds or milliseconds before the event, perform the Kegel exercise they have been diligently practicing. As they initially sense a cough or sneeze, before they reach down to tie their shoelaces, or while they are taking a brisk walk, they should first squeeze the appropriate muscles. They will minimize stress incontinence because an increased urinary outlet pressure will offset the rise in intra-abdominal pressure generated by the activity. For men predominantly dealing with urge incontinence after radiation or surgery, I recommend that when they feel the strong, sudden urge to urinate, instead of dashing to find the nearest bathroom, which may be too far away, they should pause and similarly do the exercise. In this scenario, urge incontinence is minimized through a spinal reflex that senses increased pubococcygeal muscle activity and sends out information to the bladder to cancel the involuntary bladder spasm. It is particularly useful just before high-risk activities like standing from a seated position and turning on running water.

Fluid Restriction

It may seem like an obvious suggestion to some but I will emphasize it anyway: limit fluid intake. It makes sense that drinking less fluid would result in producing less urine, which in turn means there would be less urine leaking. Many patients subscribe to the familiar myth that it is healthy to drink eight to ten glasses of water a day and they would not think of modifying this behavior after treatment. Patients may tell me that excessive fluids are required to treat constipation or that they have been instructed to take a medication with a full glass of water. These general recommendations may or may not be appropriate for many people but adhering to them will surely pronounce pre-existing urinary incontinence. It is especially important to limit certain fluids—like alcohol, caffeinated coffee, soda, and tea—and some vegetables, fruits, and herbs that have a natural diuretic effect like cranberries, watermelon, cabbage, beets, asparagus, and more. Ask your health care provider about this.

Medication

Urinary urge incontinence and urinary frequency are primarily treated pharmacologically with a class of medications called anticholinergics/antispasmodics. Anticholinergic medications, e.g. Ditropan, Vesicare, Enablex, Sanctura relax bladder muscle activity. Fortunately, these medications are much more effective against the unwanted, involuntary bladder spasms than against the vital, coordinated bladder contractions that are needed to empty urine from the bladder. The main side effect from these medications is dry mouth. Some people will complain of constipation, abdominal pain, dizziness, blurred vision, and confusion. New preparations are now available to decrease side effects that may be intolerable. Oxytrol is a patch and Gelnique is a gel that is applied to the skin. These medications are absorbed into the body directly through the skin.

Surgery

Stress urinary incontinence that does not adequately improve over time, even with pelvic floor muscle training and behavioral modification, is most successfully treated with additional surgery. The most modest surgical procedure is the injection of a bulking agent, such as collagen, into the urethra. Typically, a cystoscope is passed into the urethra just beyond the external urinary sphincter. This location is where the prostate would normally be located if it had not previously been removed with a radical prostatectomy. Using a long, flexible needle, the urologist injects the bulking agent deep to the urethral mucosal lining until it bulges inward to narrow the space and create the needed resistance. The advantages of this procedure are that it is safe, requires minimal anesthesia and surgical time, and has only a few negative side effects. The disadvantages are that it usually requires multiple treatments and needs to be repeated, and that it more often diminishes incontinence rather than making people dry or near dry. One study demonstrated that 35.2% of incontinent radical prostatectomy patients treated with collagen injection therapy were socially continent, defined in the study as totally dry or requiring no more than one pad per day. Of those men who initially became socially continent, 60.9% were socially continent after one year of follow-up, and 42.8% were at two years follow-up. A median of four separate office procedures was initially required to achieve social continence. In my experience, this treatment has lost significant popularity currently.

Urologists consider the artificial urinary sphincter prosthesis as the "gold standard." In this procedure, an inflatable cuff is positioned around the urethra through a perineal incision. A small fluid reservoir is placed under the abdominal muscles and a tiny pump is inserted into the scrotum alongside a patient's testicles. When the surgery has been completed, none of the components are visible and only the pump can be appreciated if the scrotum is felt. The cuff is normally filled with fluid so that it exerts closing pressure on the urethra. While the bladder is filling with urine, the urethral resistance minimizes urine leakage. When a man feels a significant urge to urinate, he just reaches down and squeezes the pump inside his scrotum. This activates the fluid-filled cuff to circulate its fluid into the reservoir, diminishes urethral pressure, and allows him to urinate. After three minutes, the cuff automatically refills and restores continence until the next time he squeezes the scrotal pump. The main advantage of an artificial sphincter is that it achieves the most favorable long-term continent success rates. The main disadvantage is the risk of re-operation for infection, erosion, and malfunction of the prosthesis. In one study of men who underwent insertion of an artificial urinary prosthesis after a previous a radical prostatectomy, at a mean follow-up of 7.7 years 27% used no pads, 32% used one pad/day, 15% used one to three pads/day and 25% used more than three pads per day. The re-operation rate for infection was 1.4%, prosthesis erosion was 4%, and malfunction was 25%.

A third surgical intervention for post-prostatectomy stress urinary incontinence is the bone-anchor male sling. Through a perineal incision, a mesh sling is implanted under the urethra and secured with sutures to the pubic bone. It serves as a hammock to compress the underside of the urethra. Short-term success rates of 39.5% to 90% have been reported. The risk of complications and reoperations appears to be comparable between the suburethral sling studies and the artificial sphincter studies. For mild to moderate incontinence, the bone-anchor male sling is an acceptable alternative to the "gold standard" artificial urinary sphincter. For severe incontinence, success rates and patient satisfaction rates with the sling are discouraging.

Urinary dysfunction and incontinence are significant complications of prostate cancer treatment. Radical prostatectomy is associated with higher rates of incontinence than radiation therapy. Objective rates of incontinence improve over time. When pelvic floor muscle training, fluid restriction, and behavioral modification do not satisfactorily improve stress urinary incontinence, surgical interventions are beneficial.

Prostate Cancer in HIV-Positive Patients in the Era of Highly-Active Antiretroviral Therapy (HAART)

Matthew S. Wosnitzer, MD and Franklin C. Lowe, MD, MPH, FACS

Prostate cancer is the most common noncutaneous (not skin related) malignancy and the second leading cause of cancer death in American men, with 192,00 estimated new cases and more than 27,300 deaths expected each year. While prostate screening has improved detection rates, the increased monitoring has led to earlier diagnosis in men without symptoms of the disease and, subsequently, stage migration towards localized disease.

New data from the World Health Organization (WHO) and the Joint United Nations Program on HIV/AIDS (UNAIDS) indicate that global HIV prevalence has leveled off and that the number of new infections has declined; however, 33.2 million people in 2007 were estimated to be living with HIV, 2.5 million people became newly infected, and 2.1 million people died of AIDS. Of these patients, 1.2 million Americans, including 870,000 males, were living with HIV/AIDS in the United States. More than half of all newly diagnosed HIV patients are African-American, and more than a quarter are older than forty-five years of age. Since the incidence of prostate cancer increases with age, and the risk is further increased in men of African-American descent and in immuno-compromised individuals, possibly including those with HIV/AIDS, it is expected that we will be treating prostate cancer more frequently in HIV-positive patients in the future.

Prior to the highly-active antiretroviral therapy (HAART) era that began in 1995, there were several case reports of patients with AIDS and prostate cancer who demonstrated rapid cancer progression, which was likely due to their severely-depressed immune systems and hypogonadal states, which lead to poor responses to androgen deprivation therapy. Now with the advent of HAART, HIV-positive patients with prostate cancer seem to respond to treatment similarly to patients without HIV/AIDS. The availability of HAART has led to a shift in the natural spectrum of HIV disease: It has mitigated the progression of HIV to AIDS, as well as to AIDS deaths. This has enabled HIV-positive patients to live longer and to age more normally, which allows them to get non-AIDS-defining malignancies: prostate, lung and colorectal, for example. Although several studies have identified increased incidences of some non-AIDS-defining malignancies, other studies have reported decreased incidences HAART has been suggested to be protective against non-AIDS defining malignancies, but this effect is still uncertain.

Incidence

The exact incidence of prostate cancer in HIV-infected patients is unknown. A review of the literature found available clinical and demographic data for sixty-seven cases described in case reports and another 862 described in population-based studies. Although several large population studies suggested a lower than expected prostate cancer risk in HIV-positive men during both the pre-HAART and HAART eras, other smaller studies found either similar or elevated incidences of prostate cancer in HIV-positive men compared with the general population.

A 2008 analysis of cancer incidence trends in HIV-infected patients in the United States compared the rates of all cancers among 54,780 HIV-positive patients in two multicenter prospective observational cohorts, the Adult and Adolescent Spectrum of HIV Disease (ASD) Project and the HIV Outpatient Study (HOPS) with the Surveillance, Epidemiology, and End Results (SEER) data from the National Cancer Institute. 3,550 cases of cancer were identified in the two prospective studies of HIV-positive patients; 20% were non-AIDS-defining. Between 1992 and 2003, incidence rates of Kaposi sarcoma and non-Hodgkin lymphoma declined, while there were significant increases for anal, colorectal, and prostate cancer. For the years 1992 to 1995, there were 14.7 cases of prostate cancer per 100,000 persons per year; however, from 2000 to 2003 the rate was 37.5 per 100,000 people per year. The increased incidence of prostate cancer in HIV-positive patients is most likely a reflection and result of PSA screening, because there was also a similar rise in incidence of prostate cancer in the general population during the same period from 47.4 to 60.9 cases per 100,000 persons per year.

A 2009 study found similar results in Australia. A significant decline in the incidence of prostate cancer in HIV-positive patients was observed across the period. Of note was that from 2000 to 2004, the incidence of prostate cancer was lower than that in the general population. A meta-analysis of seven studies encompassing 444,172 HIV-positive men identified a decreased risk for prostate cancer for HIV-positive men compared HIV-negative men.

Epidemiological studies of prostate cancer detection in HIV-infected patients rely upon PSA testing and rectal examination. Reports of lower prostate cancer incidences for HIV-positive men may be the result of decreased screening, although those with HIV tend to be under closer medical supervision than HIV-negative men. Also, HIV-positive men frequently have lower androgen levels; this may cause lower than expected PSA levels since normal PSA secretion is androgen dependent. This factor may decrease their likelihood that they will undergo a prostate biopsy, thereby decreasing the likelihood of having prostate cancer being detected.

Risk Factors

While the specific causes of prostate cancer have not been elucidated, there is evidence that genetics, inflammation, infection, and environmental factors seem to influence the development of the disease. Established risk factors include: family history, ethnic origin (African-American descent), and diet-related factors, such as obesity and high polyunsaturated fat intake. Increased body-mass index (BMI), which can be a result of HAART, has been consistently associated with increased risk of biochemical progression, metastasis, and fatal outcomes in prostate cancer patients. Risk also increases with the number of affected family members, with their degree of relatedness, and with the age at which they were diagnosed. Additionally age-adjusted prostate cancer mortality is 2.4 times higher in African-American men compared to white men.

In the pre-HAART era, there were several reports of HIV being associated with increased prostate cancer virulence, particularly in those who were hypogonadal at the time of their prostate cancer diagnosis. Hypogonadism is frequently found in HIV-positive males. Androgen deficiency in HIV-positive men has been associated with low CD4+ T-cell counts, more advanced disease stage, and weight loss or wasting syndrome. Hypogonadism is 20% more common in HIV-positive patients compared with age-matched healthy individuals. The etiology may be related to HIV or more likely to malnutrition. The frequent usage of testosterone supplementation and replacement therapy in HIV-positive men may account for an increased risk of prostate cancer detection due to rises in PSA levels.

The effect of HAART on decreasing cancer risk may in part be due to CD4+ T-cell counts. Other potential factors include: decreased immune activation and cytokine levels, improved immune responses unmeasured by CD4 cell count, and HAART-related suppression of cancer producing viruses. The effects of antiretroviral therapy on the hypothalamic–pituitary–gonadal axis are still poorly defined. HAART causes insulin resistance, which seems to cause a decrease sensitivity of this axis, thereby resulting in decreased testosterone secretion resulting in PSA levels being lower. The HIV-positive men being treated with HAART are less likely to undergo prostate biopsy and therefore have a lower incidence of prostate cancer than the general population.

Diagnosis

Prostate cancer screening includes digital rectal examination (DRE) and annual measurement of serum PSA level. The role of population-wide prostate cancer screening remains in question. And screening of HIV-positive patients for non-AIDS-defining malignancies, including prostate cancer, remains equally controversial. Screening practices during the PSA era, however, have caused stage migration, with increased detection of cancers of lower stages and smaller volumes. Current American Urological Association (AUA) guidelines recommend screening of all men aged forty years or older with a life expectancy greater than ten years. Baseline PSA is established at this time, which determines future screening intervals. Men at increased risk of malignancy and with a life expectancy greater than ten years (most HIV-positive patients currently have a life expectancy greater than ten years) should also begin screening at an earlier age, although no formal recommendations are available from the AUA. According to the AUA guidelines, PSA testing in patients with a serum

PSA level greater than 4.0 has a sensitivity of about 20% in contemporary series. The specificity of PSA testing is approximately 60% to 70% at this cutoff. Among men in their forties and fifties, a PSA level above the median value for age is a stronger predictor of future prostate cancer development than is family history or ethnicity. Measurement of the PSA level is a more specific test for prostate cancer in younger men compared to older men, as prostatic enlargement is less likely to confound interpretation of the estimated PSA value. Serum testosterone level should also be checked to ensure that measurement of PSA levels is accurate.

Transrectal-ultrasound-guided (TRUS) prostate biopsy is indicated in patients with an elevated PSA level or abnormal DRE findings. There are no reports in the literature suggesting increased complications from biopsy in HIV-positive patients when compared to HIV-negative individuals. Patients should refrain from receptive anal intercourse and ejaculation for at least forty-eight hours prior to a PSA test, as these could lead to transient, abnormal elevation of PSA level.

Treatment and Management

The patient's life expectancy and medical comorbidities are central in determining whether to treat prostate cancer and in choosing the optimal therapeutic approach. With the dramatically reduced life expectancies of HIV-positive and AIDS patients in the pre-HAART stage of the epidemic, physicians usually offered radiation therapy instead of radical prostatectomy as primary treatment for localized disease since life expectancy for these patients was likely less than ten years. With the widespread use of HAART and consequently extended life expectancy for HIV-positive patients, the natural history of prostate cancer in these patients seems to be similar to that in the general population. Whether HIV-positive patients respond differently to prostate cancer therapies than HIV-negative patients has to be determined. Short-term outcome analyses appear similar; however, there are no long-term follow-up reports.

Radiation therapy was shown to be efficacious with minimal morbidity in the short-term in a retrospective study of fourteen HIV-infected patients with prostate cancer, of whom two received external-beam radiotherapy, four received brachytherapy, and eight completed a combination of brachytherapy and external-beam radiotherapy. The urinary, bowel, and sexual adverse effects after treatment were found to be comparable when compared with other series of HIV-negative men. Their conclusion was that radiation therapy and brachytherapy of the prostate were not contraindicated in HIV-positive patients. An important consideration in the treatment of gay men is the potential effect of either external-beam radiation therapy or brachytherapy upon the rectum, especially if the patient engages in receptive anal intercourse.

Preoperative assessment of HIV-positive patients for consideration for radical prostatectomy should include the standard variables used in HIV-negative patients (age, stage and grade of disease, PSA level, and co-morbidities) as well as CD4+ T-cell counts, viral load, and serum albumin level. The efficacy and safety of radical prostatectomy was examined in a 2006 study in a series of five HIV-infected men (aged forty-five to fifty-nine years) with early stage prostate cancer, and moderate Gleason scores (see glossary). Three patients were receiving HAART at the time of surgery, and the median follow-up duration was twenty-six months. After radical prostatectomy, two of five patients had wound infections, one of whom required hospitalization and intravenous antibiotics. No patients progressed to AIDS during the study period, and none had biochemical recurrence during follow-up. In a comparable group we found wound infections noted in the four patients who underwent radical retropubic prostatectomy (three open, one laparoscopic) for early stage (T1c) prostate cancer. Postoperative PSA levels were undetectable in all patients, none of whom showed evidence of recurrence after a mean follow-up duration of 18.5 months. Overall, prostatectomy is well tolerated by patients with CD4+ T-cell counts greater than 500 cells per mm3 and asymptomatic HIV infection.

In our study group of sixteen patients who had various therapies for localized disease, the most recent PSA values (after a mean follow-up duration of 4.66 years) indicate their prostate cancer was controlled or stable in all patients, regardless of treatment type. Active surveillance is a reasonable option for HIV-positive patients who fulfill the criteria that are used for the general population. Repeat prostate biopsy within six months of diagnosis is the most important predictor of progression for patients on active surveillance.

In another group study of sixteen patients with HIV (mean duration of disease 8.5 years) and prostate cancer who received various treatments, all treated patients had a complete response with undetectable PSA levels and absence of tumor recurrence. No serious treatment-related adverse effects were noted. These relatively small groups indicate short-term response to therapy in HIV-positive patients with prostate cancer appears to be similar to that of the general population.

Adverse Effects of Prostate Cancer Treatment in HIV-Positive Patients

All therapies for the treatment of prostate cancer can negatively impact one's quality of life, sexual function, urinary and bowel function, as well as one's psychological state. These issues are discussed in depth in another essay in this volume. Patients, especially those on HAART, must be counseled regarding the risks of erectile dysfunction following surgical, radiation, or hormonal treatment for prostate cancer. For those undergoing surgical procedures, CD4+ counts are important because it has been shown in HIV-positive women having gynecological surgery that those with CD4+ counts less than 200 have three to four times greater complication risk than HIV-negative age and procedure matched controls. Additionally, serum albumin, a marker for nutritional status, has been associated with morbidity and mortality outcomes for those undergoing surgery with end-stage renal disease, cardiovascular disease, and numerous types of cancer as well as HIV infection. Again, gay men who engage in anal receptive intercourse need to be advised about radiation effects upon the anus and rectum for both brachytherapy and external beam radiation therapy.

With the prolonged survival of HIV-positive patients receiving highly active anti-retroviral therapy, the screening, diagnosis, and treatment of non-AIDS-defining malignancies, such as prostate cancer, now need to be addressed. All HIV-positive males over the age of forty years with a ten-year life expectancy should be screened for prostate cancer, in accordance with current recommendations of the American Urological Association for the general population. HIV-positive patients with localized prostate cancer should be offered all available treatment options. Clinical stage and grade of prostate cancer as well as HIV status and treatment history are important considerations in determining appropriate cancer therapy. Early results indicate that responses to prostate cancer therapies in HIV-positive patients are comparable to those in the general population.

Coming Out to Doctors

Darryl Mitteldorf, LCSW

The closet is a refuge, a fort, a shelter, a weapon against revelation and a way station. A closet gives time: time to ponder what to reveal, time to consider what to take out of the closet and show the rest of the world. Diagnosed with prostate cancer, men who have sex with men (MSM) are challenged with the burden of coming out to a variety of strangers, namely their doctors, who have the power to extend or harm their lives, or avoid dealing with them altogether.

A Clinical Example

Past experiences had informed Simon's expectations. During the early 1990s, Simon said he happened to let his dentist know that he was gay. Something about a discussion of an essay in a waiting-room magazine prompted the revelation. The dentist mentioned that he wasn't aware that Simon was gay. He then excused himself and left Simon alone in the chair, with the hygienist. Returning with two face shields, like clear plastic versions of a welder's mask, the dentist joked about the latest fashion accessories for dentistry and went about doing Simon's root canal. Simon wondered to himself, and over time convinced himself, that had he not mentioned that he was gay, the dentist would not have excused himself to get the facemasks. Simon said, from that moment on, he felt it was part of his life's mission to be out always, as a way to positively change the world.

Toward the beginning of 2004, at age forty-eight,

Simon presented with a positive Digital Rectal Exam (DRE), and a Gleason 8 (4+4) with six of eight positive biopsy cores (see glossary). Simon met with only one doctor, in one hospital setting, and opted to have a radical prostatectomy six weeks after diagnosis. He chose to tell his urologist that he was gay. Simon also chose to bring his long-time partner with him to pre-surgical consults. Simon introduced him as his husband.

Simon has been impotent since surgery. He says that he was surprised that he no longer has ejaculate and was not informed of this prior to surgery. In 2009, Simon's PSA once again became significant and he is currently being treated for recurrent prostate cancer.

Today, Simon spends a good deal of time in psychotherapy, talking about his feelings of regret in telling his urologist that he was a gay man. Simon says that he feels certain that his health would be no different today had he been open about his sexuality, but he has significant concern that his quality-of-life has suffered. Though he now knows that many men are impotent after a radical prostatectomy, Simon wonders if his surgeon, somehow, "acted out" in a negative fashion while performing his surgery. Simon recalls how his doctor stressed that radiation treatment might irritate the anus and make anal receptive sex unpleasant, which, today, leads Simon to think that his doctor pushed him into surgery because he is gay. Simon feels angry with himself mostly for not seeking second and third opinions. We explored issues about authorities, expectations, and disappointments, as well as self-blame and experiences of abuse.

On the other hand, I have heard wonderfully positive reports of straight doctors being quite open and eager to address their gay patients' concerns. One man who has sex with other men described his enjoyment of fisting and prostate massage, which apparently perplexed his urologist. The patient reported that the urologist readily expressed ignorance, but promised to Google the matter and learn more; and, indeed, he followed up with his patient by phone.

Options for Treatment Following Diagnosis of Prostate Cancer

Prostate cancer presents a newly-diagnosed patient with several treatment modalities, all presenting reasonably equal opportunities for extending life beyond a possibility of a cancer-caused early death. Unfortunately, all treatment modalities include significant risk of impotence and/or urinary incontinence and the certainty of diminished or eliminated ejaculate and a challenge to sex drive. One or more of these consequences are highly likely, and all patients—straight and gay—need to be fully informed as they make their treatment decisions, whether they chose surgery, radiation, or hormone treatment. Hormone therapy (androgen deprivation therapy), where testosterone is reduced to near zero, is akin to the kind of androgen punishment offered to sex offenders and, in the not-so-distant past in some countries, given to men convicted of the "crime of homosexuality."

Prostate cancer patients, particularly those in urban areas with well-chosen and affordable health insurance, have the opportunity and are well advised to consult with several doctors at different hospitals and practice settings. When diagnosed, men typically consult with a radiologist and a urologist: two doctors representing two distinct practices and staffs. Ideally, a man newly diagnosed with prostate cancer would consult with more than one urologist and radiologist, as there are several variants in treatment in each modality.

Radiation presents opportunities for brachytherapy, intensity-modulated radiation therapy (IMRT), proton beam therapy and radiation combined with androgen deprivation therapy. Surgery can be performed by urologists specializing in open radical prostatectomy, laparoscopic radical prostatectomy, and robotic laparoscopic radical prostatectomy, also with the possibility of combining androgen deprivation therapy and even follow-up radiation therapy. There are also treatments of high intensity focused ultrasound, cryotherapy, and active surveillance (watchful waiting), all requiring a consultation with a doctor specializing in one of these modalities.

A man who has sex with men will find himself meeting lots of new doctors, almost all of whom will start their consults by presuming that the patient is heterosexual. It can be a daunting challenge for a gay man to reveal his sexual orientation to these doctors. As in all coming out experiences, the gay man cannot predict how this news will be received. Moreover, these doctors are typically perfect strangers who hold significant power over the patient's medical and psychological future.

Psychotherapy with Newly Diagnosed Prostate Cancer Patients

In psychotherapy with newly diagnosed patients, we are concerned with two primary issues. First, the psychotherapist should help the patient determine how to receive the appropriate medical treatment. With prostate cancer, the consequences of treatment, such as impotence and/or incontinence, usually last years and may be permanent. Treatment must include helping the patient understand that the consequences of treatment choices can be durable and devastating.

Patients rarely acquire a clear understanding of treatment outcomes and consequences. Indeed, most all patients, gay or straight, hear the word "cancer" and hear little else that follows. Doctors generally fail to provide consultations tailored to a patient's tolerance for understanding; instead they typically provide too much or too little information during one consultation and expect the patient to digest that information over time.

For the MSM patient, understanding the consequences of treatment outcomes and morbidity within an MSM context is understandably never offered without the patient coming out. Gay patients are burdened with coming out to someone they likely have never met, and who likely has presented information as if the patient were heterosexual. The patient is burdened both with the risk and with the task of educating his doctor about gay sexual practice and eroticism. It's the rare surgeon who has sufficient time during an initial consultation to be taught how being self-identified as gay affects the patient's quality-of-life.

A psychotherapist treating a newly diagnosed prostate cancer patient must educate himself on the treatment issues, if he is not already so informed. Once knowledgeable himself, he can help the patient in three ways:

1. Educate the patient on the probable consequences of each treatment.

2. Encourage the patient to ask more detailed questions of his doctors.

3. Encourage the patient to talk with other men diagnosed with prostate cancer. Referring patients with prostate cancer to support groups like Malecare is almost always a helpful suggestion.

The second significant area in psychotherapy is the patient's regret over making an uninformed decision about treatment. Avoiding later regret is an appropriate primary goal in prostate cancer treatment choice making. Prostate cancer treatment outcomes are rarely predictable. There is no durable cure for prostate cancer and patients with reoccurrences later in life often find their way to support groups or individual therapy, complaining that they regret their initial choices.

In my practice, I have observed that it is the feeling of regret and the related neurosis that the feeling of regret highlights that pains the patient more than the intellectual wonder if a different initial treatment choice might have provided a more desirable long-term outcome. Doing all you can in the early days of prostate cancer treatment, and that you could have done no more and no better, is a proper goal towards helping to avoid later regret months and years in the future, no matter what the outcome. So, someone self-identified as a man who sleeps with men is faced with questions like: Would I regret coming out to my doctor or not? Will my treatment be different if I come out to my doctor?

Clinical Samples

Bill is a single man who was diagnosed at age fifty-three. He presented with a positive DRE and Gleason 7 (4+3). Bill works in banking. He reports satisfactory but remote relationships with various blood relatives, has a circle of supportive friends, but no significant partner. He's been out as a gay man since his early twenties, and has participated as a fundraiser for a variety of gay- and HIV/AIDS-related activities. He has told no one, beyond a neighbor, that he has been diagnosed and treated for prostate cancer.

Bill doesn't know what to make of his diagnosis. When first hearing that he had prostate cancer, Bill went home and stayed there isolating himself all weekend. He described ordering in several Chinese food meals from different restaurants, so that he would only have to deal with the deliveryman just one time. Even talking to a stranger posed a challenge for Bill in the days following his diagnosis. Now he was faced with meeting several doctors.

Bill described his consults as "chilling." He felt that

his doctors were only focused on explaining the mechanics of treatment. The surgeon recommended robotic laparoscopic surgery because he would be home in just a few days and would only need to have follow-up blood tests every few months. The radiologist explained a pain-free procedure that could be provided early in the morning, on Bill's way to work, implying that he would then go to work. He even told Bill that many of his patients enjoy meeting for breakfast and have formed new friendships as a result.

Bill wondered how to get his doctors to talk about long-term outcomes rather than the ease of treatment. He favored the idea of removing the prostate gland altogether, so he scheduled a second consultation with the surgeon.

This time, he brought in questions that he had gathered online. He also was prepared to ask if surgery would impact anal receptive sex. Bill described his question asking as simple. He asked about anal sex in between questions about anesthesia and erectile functioning. He reported that he felt better presenting his question about his future life as an anal-receptive man with little fanfare or highlight. Bill felt satisfied by his doctor's demeanor and reply, as if he had heard that question before. Bill was told that he could return to anal receptive sex after a period of healing, but that his sensations will likely be different, as he no longer will have a prostate.

For Bill, asking about anal sex was a way both to come out to his doctor and to address a concrete concern. Bill feels that he took a chance. For him, the dice rolled in his favor. But for many gay men, coming out to their doctor may prove a less-than-helpful disclosure.

John did not want to feel that he was at the mercy of anyone. A former Marine and currently a fine arts painter, he lives with his partner, a man ten years his junior who he describes as subservient. John was diagnosed at age sixty-three with a Gleason 6 in three out of twelve cores. John approached his diagnosis like a Marine assaulting a hostile beach.

He told me, "I got up one morning and put my cancer on. I went to Barnes and Noble and spent lots of time sitting in their café, reading books on prostate cancer. I bought two by what I thought to be prominent doctors and went home, stopping at Staples to buy a pack of multicolored Post-its, a pad folio with extra paper, and a set of ten pens. I had lots of writing to do."

John felt that a morbidity-laden treatment was inappropriate for him. He didn't feel that his life was being threatened by the cancer, and he felt he could live with the idea that he had cancer cells inside of him. "It's not explosive," he explained. And he enjoyed being out and an artist in New York City. Though he describes his relationship as faithful, he also enjoys meeting, flirting, and having sex with men outside of his partnership. Erections and controlling his urine are vitally important to John. He decided to find a urologist who would support his choice to maintain active surveillance.

He approached three doctors whose names he found during his research. John said that each one tried to sell him on surgery, pointing out how imperfect biopsies are in predicting the actual extent of the cancer. Each posed the idea of risk and asked John if he could live with risk. John said he resented their implication that he should trade sexual pleasure for risk reduction. John felt that his doctors didn't take time to get to know him. He felt that in each of these three consults, coming out would be fruitless.

Soon after that, John decided that all he really needed was someone who could arrange for a PSA blood test every four months. John felt that he knew enough to go it alone. But he quickly found himself napping during the hours in which he usually painted. John's partner didn't seem to mind or notice and was tolerant. Daily naps became routine. Then, Jack, a friend from England, visited, sleeping on his couch for a week while he visited New York City. Jack noticed his friend's depression and encouraged him to go for long walks with him and talk it out. John soon became aware that he felt fear that he might indeed be making the wrong decision. Since he did not come out to his doctors, he factored, he was following a choice based on less than full information.

John talked about feeling frightened. He said he didn't come out to these doctors because he felt they would not tell him about the "good stuff" in the same way they talk to straight patients. John thought that there might be a two-tier set of treatments offered and that gay men are offered inferior choices. John said that he understood that in reality his concern was mostly bankrupt. He said that doctors only make money on living patients, and that they would not care whether their money came from gay or straight patients. But he didn't come out to his doctors, and not coming out made him ruminate that he missed out on learning something that might help him live longer. John also raised an issue I had not heard of from any other gay man. Life expectancy is more and more considered in prostate cancer treatment choice-making. Men in their seventies and eighties are more and more often offered active surveillance as an option. John wondered aloud if urologists might think gay-life expectancy is less than straight-life expectancy because of HIV/AIDS. So coming out might also involve revealing a man's HIV status to his doctor. Clearly there were issues of internalized homophobia here as with the patient Simon mentioned earlier. Not infrequently the issue of internalized homophobia must be explored to enable the patient to more easily come out to his doctor.

John felt regret and a sense of helplessness, which generated anxiety-laden depression. He eventually found himself in a gay-friendly weekly support group, which helped him sort through some of his internalized homophobic reactions; he was able to consult with and be out to a fourth urologist. And John then was able to learn more about the affects of androgen deprivation therapy-related bone loss and other side effects of that treatment modality which might affect his sense of being a "dominant" man.

Some men try to manage their doctors. They don't want their doctors to feel upset and they want their doctors to see them as their best or most favorite of all patients. Some men feel that coming out would upset their health care providers and that it might compromise their treatment. These patients don't feel that being gay is a problem, but they do feel that it is a problem for others. Some men have reported their "gaydar" tells them the doctor is actually gay but closeted. Here is the risk that the patient feels that he inadvertently "outed" a gay or bisexual doctor. Patients wonder what the consequences of outing their doctor will have on their quality of treatment. I have treated one patient who thought that his surgeon might kill him during surgery rather than risk being "outed" by him. The patient survived surgery and we explored that paranoid reaction.

Some patients ascertain that coming out to their doctor would be productive and not have any negative consequences. But they wonder about the doctor's staff, particularly the office staff. Alan, a fifty-eight-year-old post-surgical patient, noted that his doctor was using an electronic records system and was typing in notes about his health and concerns. Alan said he was certain that his doctor's entire office staff read those notes, which he felt included consultations about impotence and his inability to please his partner with ejaculate or an erection during oral sex.

Alan described at length, for months on end, the barriers he felt that his urologist's hospital-based office staff put up towards him. He complained about billing errors, wrongly scheduled appointments, and even once they removed a basket of candy from the reception desk when he entered. Alan was investing a variety of psychological issues with uneasy perceptions of his doctor's staff. But he also was reporting a set of specific concrete acts that may indeed have occurred because the office staff learned that he is gay.

Summary and Recommendations

As noted, prostate cancer presents several treatment modality opportunities for most newly diagnosed patients. Treatment side effects and morbidity are experienced differently by men who have sex with men as compared to their heterosexual counterparts. Straight men do not have to come out to their doctors. There is a presumption of heterosexuality in almost all urological practices. It is rare and most welcome when I hear otherwise. In this essay, we are not looking at the biophysical aspects of treatment, but rather the challenge MSM face in deciding whether or not to disclose and discuss their sexuality in a urological consultation regarding prostate cancer.

Many MSM have had bizarre experiences with urologists who assume they are straight. One MSM prostate cancer patient told me that his doctor said he would test his post-surgical erectile functioning by asking a female nurse into the consultation room. A common statement made by urologists about diminished or no ejaculate is that there is no longer a need to wear a condom and there won't be the usual mess. Urologists seem to be mostly unaware that a gay man may be more attached to ejaculate than a straight man. Urologists also seem unaware that gay men often share or play with ejaculate as part of their sexual experience.

One startling anecdote was related by a patient who said that he was chastised by his urologist for asking one of his residents when he might be able to experience anal receptive sex after surgery. The urologist told the patient that the resident had been upset by the question.

I've met and spoken with doctors who claim that they don't have gay patients, or that they treat gay patients exactly like heterosexual patients. Many tell me that they don't ask their patients if they are gay or straight. One said, "I leave it to my patients to tell me…if they don't say anything, that's that." Another said, "I don't want to offend anyone by asking." Not one intake form or patient history that I have ever seen includes an opportunity for a man to state that he has sex with other men.

Clearly, physicians who treat prostate cancer, whether oncologists, surgeons, or radiologists, can offer treatments that prolong life itself and maintain the highest possible quality-of-life. It is also clear that prostate cancer patients are burdened with choices and challenges beyond what they ever expected life would present to them. Treatment choices are best informed by frank and interactive exchange between doctor and patient. Prostate cancer treatment presents unique sexual morbidity and poverty of outcome prognostication. Men can only make their best possible decisions if they are out to their doctors. If the doctor is not open to this, it is imperative to find another.

The burden of creating homophobic-free zones in clinical settings shouldn't have to fall on the patient. Doctors can access gay, bisexual, and transgender cultural competency via online services, such as those offered by Malecare at www.malecare.org. LGBT-appropriate intake materials can be downloaded from LGBT Cancer Project at www.lgbtcancer.org. The smallest of things, such as adding LGBT clinical brochures and magazines in waiting areas, can help put LGBT patients at ease. And including a category on intake forms for sexual orientation and/or the gender of the people the patient has sex with would be very helpful.

Doctors who themselves are men having sex with

men, or are transgendered men or women, need not feel required to be out to all patients, but should be encouraged to self-disclose to those patients who present themselves as out. At the very least, doctors should be encouraged to ask all patients if they enjoy sex with men, women, both or only with themselves as a starting point for a healthy and helpful consultation about prostate cancer treatment and associated morbidities.

What I Have Learned from Working with Gay Men Who Have Prostate Cancer

Darryl Mitteldorf, LCSW

Every man has his own list of questions about prostate cancer. Each list is unique, but all seem to carry one or more similar themes. With the hope that you will find both solidarity and surprise, here is a list of issues facing gay men, who have diagnosed with and/or treated for prostate cancer, that I have culled from narratives of hundreds of men who have attended Malecare mixed sexual orientation prostate cancer groups, uniquely gay male support groups, as well as online and in person individual consultations.

1. Coming out as a prostate cancer victim and/or survivor revisits the experience of coming out as a gay man.

Cancer victims/survivors often ask themselves questions such as: "Why do I have cancer?" "Can I be cured?" "Will I survive?" "How do I get past my fears?" "Which people can I tell about my cancer, its side effects, and my feelings about all these things without being hurt, humiliated, or abandoned?" These appear to bring up questions that gay men often ask themselves when coming out, such as "Why am I gay?" and so on. Coming out as a cancer victim/survivor also rekindles emotional memories that color a man's coming out as a man with prostate cancer. Unpleasant feelings re-emerge: feelings of numbness, fear, depression, and confusion.

But for many men, the same coping and navigation skills that they developed in coming out as gay can help them to come out as a person with prostate cancer. It's not surprising that gay men in groups of mixed sexual orientation cancer survivors often mentor straight men in sharing the diagnosis with friends, family, and care providers.

That's not to say every gay man diagnosed with prostate cancer is ready and able to be out as a cancer victim/survivor instantly. Indeed, feeling forced and compelled to come out as a cancer survivor is comparable to being bullied. It is always better that a man comes out in his own way and in his own time.

Gay men should follow their gut instincts and decide for themselves when they are ready to open the cancer closet door and come out. It may take some men more time than might seem reasonable to others; but only they can prepare themselves to work through the thoughts, fears, and emotions that have kept them silent about their diagnosis. What all gay men should know is that being out as gay men makes them better prepared to come out as a cancer survivors.

2. Sexuality varies from one gay man to another: Each individual has different tastes, fantasies, and practices when it comes to sex.

Gay sexual practices often get lumped together. It's like saying that all men who are athletic enjoy all kinds of sports. Some do, but most of us enjoy one or just a few activities. Gay men know this, but clinicians often do not. Without a frank and precise discussion of your individual sexual practices, your doctor and caregivers won't really have a clue about your concerns.

For many heterosexuals, gay sex is often equated with anal sex. They fail to recognize the play, the kissing, the affection, and the mutual masturbation, among other things, that go on between same-sex couples. Being frank and precise becomes one of the tools that gay men must use when talking about sexual side effects and prostate cancer.

Like it or not, gay men are almost always burdened with having to be their doctors' gay sex instructors.

For example, some men may find post-treatment ejaculate reduction a bonus. Some guys like the fact that there is no mess after orgasm. But some men enjoy ejaculate—the taste, the scent, and the opportunity to play with it.

Gay men in group settings can be most helpful to each other when using tolerance and understanding of various styles and preferences in the sexual arena. There is no one-way to enjoy love, sex, and sensual expression. With respect for the individual's desires and enjoyments, we each should provide a more accepting group experience for us all.

3. Gay men often struggle with low incomes and health insurance concerns just like everyone else.

Many in the straight world think that all gay men are wealthy; that they don't have children, are super creative, and that they draw on the "gay network" for jobs from other gay men. The truth is that gay men struggle with the same economy and job market as everyone else. Indeed, higher rates of depression and homophobia might point to lower job opportunities and higher rates of unemployment.

For gay prostate cancer patients, money becomes critical around health care. And it's not just single men. Gay men in relationships continue to struggle to find insurance through or for their partners, so some gay couples are paying for two health insurance policies where straight married couples would be paying for just one.

Gay men with pre-existing conditions such as HIV/AIDS often find themselves burdened with additional annual medications, tests, and consultation fees when faced with advanced prostate cancer treatment, such as androgen deprivation therapy. Further, gay couples where both men are diagnosed with prostate cancer face financial burdens and employment struggles even more so.

4. Gay men suffer stress from homophobia and gender-phobia in clinical settings.

How many times have you entered a doctor's office or hospital waiting room and found a copy of a gay publication? I bet hardly anyone has. How many times have you struggled to find the words "partner" or "bisexual" or "gay" listed on an intake or new patient form? It is a rare occurrence. And how many times have doctors presumed you were straight and presented issues around health-related side effects as if you were straight?

Gay men struggle to know who to tell and who not to tell that they are gay. Do we tell the nursing staff, the doctor, the X-ray technician, or the social worker? Sometimes gay men ask themselves, what difference will it make?

It's not easy to figure out whom to tell in a hospital or doctor's office, but there are some caregivers who you simply must tell: your doctor, for one. You need to feel completely comfortable sharing symptoms and asking questions about treatments and consequences. You need to feel open about sharing concerns of all sorts with the one or two people who are now in your life for the sole purpose of keeping you alive. Make sure that your family, friends, and partners are afforded the same rights and access as might be the case for a straight person. And you need to feel assured that all of the clinical staff—nurses, technicians, and secretaries—treats you without prejudice.

No gay man should worry about holding his lovers had during a clinical visit or kissing his partner just before a procedure.

Stress from clinical-setting homophobia exists everywhere, but it can be diminished by early discussions with your doctor. Come out and talk about issues relating to your sexual orientation as soon as possible. Build confidence in yourself and reduce the discomfort that your well-intentioned doctor may well experience by talking freely and frankly.

Don't hesitate to be open and friendly with your nurses. During hospital stays, bring a box of donuts for each of the three nursing staff shifts. You may meet a nurse who objects to homosexuality or offers to pray for you, but most nurses, in my experience, will keep their prejudices at bay if faced with a friendly man in their care. Stress reduction is in your hands. You won't be able to completely remove the stress of homophobia, but you can get the upper hand and focus on the health care issues that face you today.

5. For some gay couples, both partners may be diagnosed with prostate cancer and therefore face unique realities.

Malecare continues to be the only national nonprofit that addresses the concerns of gay couples where both men are diagnosed with prostate cancer. Rarely are both men diagnosed at the same time, but when they are, we often see that each man may choose different paths for his own treatment

Aside from their financial concerns, gay couples with prostate cancer face unique questions that, if discussed, can lead to an even stronger and more love-filled partnership. Chats about treatment choices, urinary incontinence, impotence, and the different ways we think about life and death are all important conversations that may strengthen a relationship.

6. Gay men experience ejaculate and erection envy post-treatment.

Impotence and incontinence are on the table for almost all post-radical prostatectomy patients for some period of time, if not forever. Playing with each other's erections and enjoying the taste, scent, and feel of each other's ejaculate are pleasures uniquely shared by gay men. When one man suffers incontinence, impotence, and/or an elimination of his ejaculate after surgery, some may feel they are missing out.

The healthier partner is often envious of the post-surgery partner (whose erections are compromised as a result of treatment) who gets to play with the healthy man's more fully erect penis and/or his more plentiful ejaculate. Conversely, the partner who may have suffered more deleterious side effects is often envious of the partner whose sexual apparatus is more fully functioning.

As noted, envy can be difficult to work through. Learning about relationship-building from men who have experience often helps, which is why talking about these problems in a group of gay men diagnosed with prostate cancer is so important.

7. Bisexual men may present themselves as heterosexual and may not be willing to disclose their sexuality when present with their partners or spouses.

More and more we see straight-appearing men who are secretly enjoying sex with other men showing up in our support groups. They mostly participate in our online support groups. These are men who are living in straight marriages or dating women but secretly have active sex with men. When they find themselves diagnosed with prostate cancer, they feel that their lives are challenged. How much longer will they live? What will the remainder of their lives be like? Is it now or never to be out about their sexual desires? Some men use their prostate cancer diagnosis as an opportunity to jump-tart themselves into honesty, openness, and freedom.

There are many reasons for a man to stay closeted, so in any gay support group it's important to welcome these men who have shown the courage to attend a gay men's group, even when they struggle to self-identify as gay.

8. Transgender women (MTF) are equally susceptible to prostate cancer.

Transgender women should be encouraged to ask for prostate cancer tests, such as digital rectal exams and prostate specific antigen (PSA) blood tests. Sadly, most transgender women with prostate cancer in our online groups are facing advanced stage diagnosis. We don't really know why, but it might be because of missed opportunities for early diagnosis. Prostate cancer in this respect is gender neutral. It falls to the transgendered woman to ask for tests that her doctors may otherwise not offer.

9. Gay men prefer doctors who have experience answering questions from gay patients.

It is no surprise that the best clinical experiences occur where frank, safe, and open discussion is available. That's not because a doctor is gay or straight. Doctors offering the best clinical consultations are those who are not afraid to hear the questions their patients might ask. Like all people, doctors may not ask particular questions because they are uncomfortable with a particular issue.

Doctors are more likely to discuss gay-relevant issues when they have had opportunities to interact with gay patients. When you have an initial consultation with your doctor, allow him or her time to ask you about your life. If the doctor has not asked about your sexuality, then it is appropriate to ask politely why they didn't ask. Did they presume that you are heterosexual? Perhaps they understood that you are gay, but were afraid to learn more about you. In either case, it's important that you as patient do your best to open the dialogue with your doctor.

Prostate cancer is a disease where treatment choices affect lifestyle. Being able to talk about your sex life is critical for your best care.

10. Androgen deprivation therapy has a history of punishment for the gay community.

Most of us know of the history of forced androgen deprivation therapy on gay men within the criminal justice system. In the United Kingdom, computer scientist Alan Turing, famous for his contributions to mathematics and computer science, was a homosexual who chose to undergo chemical castration in order to avoid imprisonment in 1952. Approximately eighty countries still list homosexuality as a punishable offense. And the "conversion therapy" movement sometimes includes chemical castration as a therapy to help a gay man become straight.

It is therefore no surprise when gay men balk a little more than straight men when offered androgen deprivation therapy. How threatening is it for a man who struggled to be free, open, and happy as a man who enjoys sex with men to be told that he can survive cancer only by agreeing to a life of little to no sexual desire?

There are many challenges gay men with prostate cancer face that are unique to them as a group. It's wonderful to know that the gay community no longer faces prostate cancer alone. Online and in-person support groups bring gay men with prostate cancer together, thus helping to create changes in attitudes, behaviors, and emotions through dialogues with other gay men who are going through or have been through what they are experiencing.

A Straight Urologist Discusses Working with Gay Men Diagnosed with Prostate Cancer

Franklin C. Lowe, MD, MPH, FACS

All patients, whatever their sexual preferences (homosexual, heterosexual, lesbian, bisexual, or transgender), want to be treated with respect and compassion by their physicians. They all want their physicians to be able to communicate openly about their conditions and the implications of the treatments.

Unfortunately, open communication between gay patients and their heterosexual physicians can be inhibited and stilted because of their underlying personal feelings and sentiments. It is not uncommon for the gay patient to be concerned about homophobic attitudes on the part of the physician (who is simply a representative of society as a whole); therefore, they can be reluctant and reticent to discuss their homosexual life. On the other side of the desk, many physicians are reluctant and inhibited to discuss lifestyle and sexual issues with patients in general and with gay patients in particular. Sexual history is often likely to be omitted in intake medical histories by most physicians. It is unfortunate that many heterosexual physicians have inherent biases, prejudices, and religious convictions against homosexuality that interfere with the doctor-patient relationship.

As a heterosexual urologist who has treated a large number of gay patients, I have actively tried to make my homosexual patients feel comfortable about being gay. I feel that I need to address their underlying assumptions and concerns that, as a heterosexual doctor, they may assume I am negatively judgmental and homophobic. Most importantly, I try to convey that I am open and accepting of LGBT people. Usually, during the time we are discussing their marital status/partnerships, I frequently mention the problems that my lesbian niece has had with her frequently changing legal marital status in California, going from being illegal, to being legal, to being annulled, to being remarried, and currently being constitutionally challenged.

A major factor in promoting open and successful dialogue between the gay patient and his physician is the ability of the doctor to listen and to hear the patient's concerns. Attentive listening is imperative in fostering a productive doctor-patient relationship. Being an active and engaged listener is respectful of the patient and fosters mutual trust. Listening to the patient's story becomes the first step in the therapeutic process. It helps to create a safe environment in which patients can share their intimate feelings.

Being compassionate and sympathetic are essential features of the doctor-patient relationship. Heterosexual physicians need to understand the complex and additional anxieties that a gay patient has living in a heterosexually-dominated society. Recognizing the challenges that come with being gay enables physicians to respond to the particular needs of the gay patient. Compassion for the gay patient comes with an understanding of the patient as a complete human being.

Openness on the part of the physician is essential in creating an effective dialogue. This enables the physician to obtain a complete and accurate history, including lifestyle and sexual practices. Obtaining an accurate history is the most important factor in the evaluation and management of a patient's condition. Knowledge about these issues is extremely important in discussing and choosing treatment options for a gay man with prostate cancer.

An additional issue to be addressed is the physical

examination of the genitalia and the rectum. Many physicians overlook this part of the physical exam because they have been inadequately trained to evaluate this part of the anatomy and are uncomfortable with palpation of the sexual organs. Therefore, it is common for urologists and proctologists to be the only physicians who do thorough examinations of the male genitalia and prostate. Societal inhibitions have led to this reality. Unfounded concerns of physicians regarding the risks of occupational exposure to viral illnesses prevent many doctors from wanting to examine and treat gay men. From the patients' perspective, all men, whether gay or heterosexual, find the examination of their genitals and prostate embarrassing and uncomfortable. It is imperative that the physicians make their patients feel as relaxed and comfortable as possible.

At the time of diagnosis of prostate cancer, the urologist must be supportive, sympathetic, and compassionate. Because this discussion is very emotionally challenging, it is certainly beneficial for the patient to have his partner or another person present at the time of this discussion. In addition to emotional support for the patient, the partner or friend has a better chance of recalling what the patient has been told. This discussion is clearly the most difficult time for a patient for three reasons. First, the cancer is a threat to his life. Second, the treatments are a threat to his manhood because sexual dysfunction is a common side effect of these treatments. Third, the treatments are also a threat to his social well-being because of potential problems with urinary control.

Each treatment option needs to be fully explained and reviewed with the patient so that he can understand the risks and benefits of each therapy. Most importantly, the issues concerning cancer control, urinary control, and sexual function need to be discussed with a complete understanding of the patient's personal life. All the available treatments can have deleterious effects upon sexual function, including penile length, prostate sensation, erectile function, ejaculation, and libido. Knowledge about whether the patient engages in anal-receptive intercourse is an important issue when discussing radiation treatments, either external beam or brachytherapy (radioactive seed implantation) to the prostate because proctitis and anal stenosis are potential complications of these therapies. Radical prostatectomy frequently causes decrease in sexual sensation from the removal of the prostate, penile shortening as well as diminished rigidity when erectile function returns. Banking sperm for the future is an important issue to raise with any man undergoing treatment for prostate cancer, particularly younger men, but it is typically overlooked when working with gay men.

The urologist, when giving advice to their prostate cancer patients, needs to find an acceptable balance between respecting a patient's autonomy and guiding the patient's decisions in terms of what is in their best interest based on their expressed values and long-term goals. This can only be achieved if the urologist has a complete understanding of the patient's personal life, social environment, work situation, and sexual practices. Without having established open communication with the patient about these issues, the urologist will not be able to provide the most appropriate assessment of what are potentially the best options for the individual patient.

Thus, the key aspect in the successful management and treatment of gay patients is the development of a strong doctor-patient relationship; this relationship is based upon the establishment of open communication between them. This can only occur if the physician is non-judgmental and accepting and the patient is comfortable with sharing. It is imperative that the physician asks about a person's sexual life. And it is equally important that the patient respond as honestly as he is able. If the doctor doesn't ask, then it is imperative that the patient open up the dialogue. If the physician is unable or unwilling to have this kind of open discussion, it behooves the patient to find another doctor.

Part Two

Experiential Section

Active Surveillance/Anxious Surveillance: A Gay Man Chooses Watchful Waiting

"Mark Red"

My Choice

Active surveillance isn't for everyone. There is a reason people ruefully refer to it as "anxious surveillance." It means living with the worry that your health could take a turn for the worse, that you could in fact be endangering your life. So why choose active surveillance? Because there are cases when it is a reasonable decision. And just because one is not choosing treatment this month does not mean the decision won't change as conditions change. Dr. Peter Scardino of Memorial Sloan Kettering Cancer Center in New York City has written that men with slow-growing cancers may not need immediate treatment. The operative word here is "immediate." Some people who choose this option have surgery or radiation within two years of first choosing active surveillance. Some don't need it at all. By the time this essay is read, I have no idea where I will be with regard to treatment, but as of this writing, I have been on active surveillance for seventeen months since first being diagnosed with prostate cancer. It is a decision I made even though I was fifty-five years old when I was first diagnosed. In the past, I understood that doctors only recommended what used to be called "watchful waiting" for men over seventy who might not recover well from surgery and who might well die of some other cause before prostate cancer-caused death.

I am fifty-seven now, and I haven't had surgery,

radiation, or any other treatment for prostate cancer. Thus I have not had to live with the potential side effects of those treatments. And in the seventeen months since my first diagnosis, my test results seem to show a remission of the prostate cancer. Where there was once a palpable tumor, my doctor can now feel nothing. My PSA numbers have trended downward rather than upward. My follow-up biopsy showed no cancer cells in the core samples taken. My first biopsy came back with a Gleason score of 6 and a clear sign of cancer cells. Six months later, in my second biopsy, they found no cancer cells. They did find the least aggressive kind of Prostatic Intraepithelial Neoplasia (PIN) cells (a pathologically identifiable condition thought to be a possible precursor of prostate cancer) in one core at low levels; these are abnormal cells in the prostate that appear in more than half of all men over fifty. If aggressive PIN cells are found, there is a higher chance that cancer will be present. But low-grade PIN cells are the least likely to develop into cancerous cells. After my second biopsy, my PSA numbers went down. Three months after that they went down again. I won't say I am in remission. I know that a biopsy is an inaccurate tool. Nor is a PSA number an absolute indicator of prostate cancer. My doctor can no longer feel the small tumor that had been present before. For the moment, I am what my doctor called "a poster boy for active surveillance." But that could change any time, which is why the surveillance is active. I get a PSA test every three months.

Sometimes I suffer from the discomfort of prostatitis (see glossary); when I feel that pain late at night, it is easy to let my mind run riot with fear and worry. The greatest side effect of active surveillance is living with the anxiety that the cancer might become aggressive and that the discomfort I experience from prostatitis might be cause for alarm. When I told friends that active surveillance was my course of action, they were shocked. First, they weren't sure it was the right course of action (or as I say, inaction) and then, given my history of hypochondriacal paranoia, they didn't believe I could do it. It is true that, since making this decision, I have had severe anxiety attacks that have kept me awake at night. Sometimes the anxiety has kept me from being able to focus on work. But I would rather live with the anxiety than with the potential side effects of prostate cancer treatment. And as near as my doctors can tell, at the moment, I am cancer free, or maybe more accurately stated, there is no detectable cancer.

A year before I was diagnosed, two friends of mine had been diagnosed with prostate cancer; one chose surgery, the other chose seed implant radiation treatment. I was with them through their decision-making process. I had learned a good deal about prostate cancer before it became an immediate concern for me. Oddly, the month before I was diagnosed, I started to learn even more about prostate cancer because at work I had been assigned to write brochures for a major cancer center seeking to publicize their urology department. Despite the preparation of being with my friends through their processes and reading about cancer treatments for my work, it still came as a punch in the gut that left me gasping for breath and dizzy with fear when I received my own diagnosis of prostate cancer.

I wasn't expecting this. My PSA level was still relatively low at 2.75. But my primary care physician, a gay man himself, noticed that it had more than doubled in two years. I was told that a doubling rate suggests an aggressive cancer. I set up an appointment with a urologist for further examination. Once again, I was fortunate to find a good urologist who was also a gay man, who, having felt something suspicious via a digital rectal exam, arranged a biopsy and delivered the bad news.

I was a fifty-five year old single gay man in relatively good health, but I felt that the "bad news" marked the end of my love life, despite evidence to the contrary from my

145

two friends who had been treated the previous year. Both of them had good outcomes in terms of being cancer free and being able to perform with their partners. It didn't matter to me. I went into a total depression, and I struggled to keep from throwing myself into compulsive sexual hook-ups. I believed that my love life and sex life were virtually coming to an end. I felt the need to have as much sex as possible before treatment because I was afraid that after treatment I would no longer be able to have sex and that I would be less desirable.

I was extremely fortunate that a third man I knew, through my synagogue, was not only a PCa survivor, but also a medical social worker active in the survivor community. He introduced me to Malecare's Gay Men's Prostate Cancer Support Group, and I am profoundly grateful. I found a place to express my fears with men who understood them. I listened to their experiences as a guide for my choices. It was a place of shared grief, fear, and also laughter and strength. Once again, I felt fortunate to live in New York City, where there is a group like this. I felt held and supported emotionally by this group of men who all had gone through what I was going through. Sometimes the meetings left me feeling hopeful, but sometimes it left me feeling more anxious, since some men related horror stories that were not pleasant to imagine in my future. Some of the issues discussed in the group triggered other demons of mine: I am in a 12-step program for sexual compulsion. Like many gay men socialized into a world of casual sex, I got lost in Internet hook-ups and anonymous encounters despite my own deeper values. I had come to understand that rather than seeking sex for meaningful connection, I was using it to avoid feelings and issues in my life with which I wasn't comfortable. Facing a disease that struck at the heart of my sexual sense of self triggered an almost overwhelming urge to have as much sex as possible, whether it was a healthy expression of my sexuality or not.

I realized that acting out sexually would be a way of avoiding my fear of mortality, my anger with feeling powerlessness, and my loneliness.

Because many of the men in the support group face problems with erectile dysfunction, it is often an important topic of discussion, so sometimes there would be discussions about the use of prostitutes to maintain regular sexual connection and keep the blood flowing, as it were. For me, this was triggering. When I say triggering, I mean that it led to the desire to act out sexually; that is, to use sexual behavior to avoid feeling the fear, anxiety, and loneliness I was experiencing. For me, healthy sexual expression is about me feeling both physical and emotional intimacy with another and with my own center. Acting out sexually for me was all about numbing myself to the pain. And a diagnosis of prostate cancer is the perfect excuse any sexually compulsive man could need to get lost in a stupor of sexual activity. To add to my anxiety, around the same time that I was diagnosed I became unemployed. To say that it was hard work during this time to stay sexually sober, emotionally balanced, and motivated is an understatement. So I am grateful not only for the support of the group of men at St. Vincent's Hospital in New York City but also to the men and women of Sexual Compulsives Anonymous, who were there with me, and continue to be there for me, every day of this part of my journey. If compulsive sexuality is something you think might be an issue for you, you can go to the SCA website to learn more about it: www.sca-recovery.org.

Taking Action

I stayed in the gay men's prostate cancer group for about a year as I went through my options, listening to the varied stories and receiving emotional support. In my first meeting I met a man who had chosen active surveillance.

He was in his seventies and his cancer had not progressed in several years. He was the only man in the group who had made that choice. My friends, mentioned earlier, were convinced I should choose one of the treatment options available, as each was convinced of the efficacy of what he had chosen, as well as the skill of his doctors. But everyone, from my friends to the members of the support group, was ready to support me in my decision because every one of these men knew that there are many ways to go in response to a diagnosis of prostate cancer; and for each of us it is an individual decision we have to make and live with.

Having a large support system was one reason I was able to make this choice. But I wouldn't have made it without hearing from two doctors at different major hospitals that in my case it was a viable choice. My first biopsy revealed a Gleason score of 6, cancer had only been found in one core out of seven on the right side, and then less than 2%. On the left side, they found PIN cells. My urologist described my prostate cancer as "indolent." It meant that it was not, as far as they could tell, aggressive. It meant that I didn't need to rush to make a decision about the course of action or treatment.

I had the requisite MRIs and bone scans. Nothing had spread outside the capsule of the prostate gland, and from what they had found, there was very little to spread. I know that a biopsy is the proverbial needle in a haystack, except the needle is in the doctor's hands and he is sticking into you a dozen or more times at different sites in a very sensitive place to say the least. It is not a foolproof or exact science. I learned that many men who had a Gleason score of 6 prior to surgery, on full examination of the removed prostate when it was possible to exam the entire gland, were reclassified with a higher score. Knowing this meant the situation could be more serious than the urologist suggested.

I did due diligence. I met with three surgeons and two radiologists. I took a friend with me to each meeting. In one of the first meetings I had with a surgeon, he actually suggested that active surveillance was a possibility for me. And he said that if it were what I chose, he would want to do another biopsy in six months, taking more samples than in the last biopsy. I didn't relish the idea of another biopsy, since I was in quite a bit of discomfort after the first one for almost three months. But another biopsy was certainly less invasive than full out surgery.

I read several studies of men who chose active surveillance, and the so-called "algorithm for eligibility," which helps to determine one's viability for being able to consider active surveillance. The following conditions should be in play to consider active surveillance:

1. Gleason score of 6 or less.
2. PSA less than 10.
3. Fewer than three biopsied cores involved.
4. Rectal digital exam score between T1c – T2a stages of the cancer.

I was well within these parameters and thus clearly a very good candidate for active surveillance. Sloan Kettering also has a nomogram that you can find on their website at http://www.mskcc.org/mskcc/html/10088.cfm. If you have your own information, you can enter it to see where you are on the scale and whether or not you are a candidate for active surveillance. Then, of course, talk it over, a lot. Once I understood this was a possible choice, I read about a study in which men diagnosed with this low level of prostate cancer made lifestyle changes regarding diet that resulted in a significant percentage of them seeing a drop in their PSA scores.

This was enough for me. I read the literature. I figured radical changes were better than a radical prostatectomy. I cut out red meat. I cut out all dairy fats. I cut back on sugar. I added soy to my diet in a major way. I ate tofu almost every day, soy cereal, soymilk, broccoli, broccoli sprouts, and pomegranate seeds in soy-based cereal with soymilk. I ate only organic chicken, turkey, or salmon for animal protein. I put tomato sauce on something every day. I drank green tea and wheat grass juice. I also added supplements: Zyflamend, vitamin D, green tea extract, soy isoflavones, and anti-oxidants of many varieties.

I attended lectures on nutrition and cancer. Some of what I was doing was recommended. Some was not recommended. And some was actively discouraged. For example, there are negative effects to eating so much soy. I just kept at it. And I did something else not in the literature: I saw a faith healer whom I knew was someone who had good results with other people. Everyone must choose for himself; I'm reporting everything I did. And quite frankly, I did so much that I am not prepared to say what worked and what didn't. But for the moment, something was working and I wasn't questioning anything.

Meanwhile, my prostate had been traumatized by the experience of the biopsy and was occasionally inflamed. I developed bacterial prostatitis. It was quite uncomfortable. The pain would wake me up in the middle of the night. I would then be unable to go back to sleep, uneasy and unsure of whether I had made the right decision.

I had chosen a surgeon from the several I had interviewed, and while I had already begun my lifestyle changes, he had me undergo another test: an endorectal MRI, which indicated that the cancer was extremely small and localized (it hadn't escaped the prostate capsule). The imaging from this test, along with the image from an ultrasound exam, would guide my next biopsy to what appeared to be the most suspicious areas. I had my second biopsy six months after the first biopsy. The doctor took more core samples than had been taken in my first one, but it was no less traumatic, though this time I very wisely took anti-anxiety medication before undergoing the procedure.

I've stated the result of this biopsy before, but it was a complete shock to me. It showed no cancer. Nothing. Nada. Zip. In one core they found PIN cells of the least aggressive variety. I was both totally happy and completely untrusting of the result. After all, it is needle in a haystack. He could have missed the cancer, since it is so small. I refused to celebrate and remained suspicious of the result. I actually felt like it would be inviting the universe to zap me if I did. The surgeon said that whatever it is I was doing, keep doing it.

However, when it came to my strict diet, I won't pretend that keeping it up is easy. I won't say I have been perfect. I love cheese and it was hard to give it up. Soy Parmesan just doesn't cut it. While sugar is like pouring gasoline on a fire for cancer, I needed my chocolate. After all, I wasn't having any sex, and I needed some substitute comfort food. I was just careful not to overdo it.

It helped to have a community of friends who supported me in my decision and who didn't try to take me off my rather strict diet. One of these friends lives on the West Coast, and he bore the brunt of my late-night calls, talking me down from anxiety attacks. Given the uncertainty of making this decision, I did not tell my parents. They are in their eighties, and this is not a decision that they would have been able to understand, nor deal well with emotionally. I did not need the pressure of their anxiety on top of my own substantial load.

Over the next three months, while I waited for my prostate to calm down after the trauma of the second biopsy, I experienced the same discomfort of pain that would wake me at night; and during the day I felt like I had to urinate a dozen times. I was completely convinced the biopsy results were faulty. Both antibiotics and anti-inflammatory medication were prescribed and they helped calm things down. And I would, on occasion, take half a Xanax (Alprazolam) to get through the night.

In March, eleven months after my original diagnosis, I had a follow-up PSA test, and the results showed my PSA had dropped from the initial high of 2.75 down to 1.75. Three months later, it had dropped yet again to 1.48. It was a clear downward trend. The next time I saw the surgeon, the results of the digital rectal exam were also good.

It is now four months since my last PSA test. My next appointment with the surgeon is in five months. But I have been uncomfortable this month again and have had symptoms that could be either prostatitis or a resurgence of the prostate cancer. I had a PSA test last week and the numbers had gone up slightly. But given my history, my surgeon prescribed antibiotics for the presumptive diagnosis of bacterial prostatitis. After two weeks on the meds, I am no longer experiencing the pain and discomfort. When I finish the course, I'll have another PSA test and see how things go after that.

Life Goes On

In the meantime, my dating life has been a train wreck. Here I am facing a disease that keeps me up at night with worry that it could kill me, and yet I'm still thinking about sex and love. After a biopsy, one typically ejaculates blood in the semen for up to three months. Not exactly something I want to explain to a potential bedmate. But two months after the second biopsy, I started dating again. I face all the issues a single, older gay man deals with and sometimes it is discouraging; another excuse for acting out that I resist. But I haven't lacked for dates with men of quality. Eventually I have to tell them what's going on. Not unlike men who must disclose their HIV status, I have to tell a potential mate something that may affect the sexual experience and the relationship (assuming it continues and gets serious). Choosing the point at which to do that is difficult. But relationships require honesty and I truly want to find a life partner for the years remaining, which could be another thirty or more. And if it doesn't start on that solid rock of emotional honesty and intimacy it won't last, and it won't be the relationship I really want. I admit it, I want to get married, and I want my photo in the New York Times! And someday, with or without my prostate, I know I will.

A Method for Identifying the Best Doctor and Treatment for Prostate Cancer

John Dalzell

Men with prostate cancer basically experience their initial diagnosis in a similar way. Uncertainty creeps into his every pore. Then his questions typically start with asking about life expectancy: Is this going to be a death sentence? Eventually, a critical question surfaces: Whom will he go to for help? These questions happened to me, too, when I was forty-eight. I sat down with my doctor to learn about my prostate cancer. "You certainly are unusual," he said, peering deep into my eyes. "You have no family history of the disease. You're a nonsmoker and a nondrinker, and eight months ago you had a normal PSA." Still in eye-lock, I whispered, "Go figure, sometimes it just happens." Lightly laughing, we nodded in agreement. "And it does just happen sometimes," he said warmly. He suggested that most men go for advice to three to four different specialists. They then decide what treatment would be best for them. Each doctor offers his own medical technique, along with possible side effects. However, what my doctor could not suggest was how to choose the best treatment that could deliver the best physical outcome for me.

That decision had to be more than a simple matter of compare and contrast between physicians and medical techniques. After all, this cancer was about my body and its future capabilities. It was not a grocery store list. I knew at the start of my cancer diagnosis that the decision to choose the best medical intervention was going to be mine alone.

That was clear. So were my choices: surgical removal of the prostate, which would be done traditionally with the scalpel or the updated surgical version, using robotics. Radiation therapy was another option, chemotherapy was not considered advisable for my early diagnosis; and there was, also for me, the choice of watchful waiting, which was a wait and see what happens method. In part, making the best decision did mean considering the obvious. I needed to find out the pluses and minuses associated with each procedure. That was easy. Rather like adding two and two. But even Freud suggested that we can't imagine our own death. How then could I imagine any kind of world associated with the loss of my erections? What exactly are all of the factors that could change my relationship with my male partner even beyond our sexual activities? And when do all of these events show up after my radiation treatment or surgery? Freud was correct, I could not cope nor could I really imagine what sex and my relationship would be like in the future. I just could not see it.

I desperately needed grounding, some kind of architecture to build my thoughts and feelings around. I called upon my training in research, statistics, and work within the medical field and medical education to find out what the best way to decide what might be best for me. Even though my Gleeson score was low (3+3) and my physician gave me several months to make a decision, my head was racing to make choices. I decided that extending life as long as possible was my primary concern. Everything else would be secondary.

Sure, I knew before scheduling any appointment that each doctor establishes different levels of trust. Each would offer his medical approaches and present different outcomes. But I wanted some level of certainty about my decision-making. I wanted conversations beyond just going on trust and cause and effect medical outcomes. So how I could best obtain this assurance became the first question.

Fortunately, having no mental models for making life decisions was not unfamiliar turf for me nor for many gay men. As gay people we often go along unguided by others, making personal decisions in our lives. Unfortunately, many straight people in our families and communities actively avoid discussing or offering models to us on how we should love, live, raise children, and nurture ourselves. They just don't talk deeply about our lives with us. The result is that we often learn to relate to our bodies, partners, and selves through self-reflection and experience without the assistance of our family and community. We often have to figure it on our own. At midlife, I was familiar with the lack of road signs telling me where I am and where to go next for help. Maturity and life experiences also made me an active information-processer on this journey. My path takes a specific kind of thinker. I was not interested in learning how the medical procedures differed. I wanted to know about something all physicians had in common. I basically wanted to know: How do these cancer specialists think and learn today? Focusing on their active thinking and learning process offered me "up to the minute" research data about what method would allow me to live the longest.

My investigation used the following assumptions:

A skilled surgeon or radiologist would be someone who has done his/her procedure for eight years or longer. That time frame led to the conclusion that a physician doing the procedure long enough had developed a high skill level acquired by simple repetition of the procedure. In other words, they had done the medical technique "hundreds of times."

One major problem with these assumptions is that specialists are human and have knowledge limitations. Not all specialists agree on what procedure is safest and offer what they believe to be the best chance for a healthy recovery.

I therefore needed to develop questions that moved

across specialty boundaries. I asked each specialist to compare what he/she knew of the other medical specialist's procedural strengths and weaknesses. So my next question became: How was I going to address a medical topic that was new to me? I knew that doctors rely on "decision making trees" and medical research. Basically, they make predictions based on the research literature in their area of medical specialty area, which is at the top of the decision tree. All I needed to do was ask about the most important research studies in their field, radiology, or surgery. Then I could ask the doctors to compare the weaknesses and strengths of the medical procedure they recommended with that of other physicians' specialties. For instance, I would ask the physician to discuss what was known of radiology outcomes and its limits. Then I would ask the radiologist about his research area and what was known about surgical outcomes.

Asking each treating physician about his knowledge of the strengths and weaknesses of recent studies in the field gave me access to the physician's thinking and why one method might be better than another, beyond the grocery list of treatment side effects and outcomes. I now had a doorway to choosing the best method based on the doctors' opinions. So I decided to talk about the research in each of the fields, with a quick overview of the specialist's particular technique, asking about how many days out of work I might expect, what side effects were likely, and so forth.

I needed, however, more insight before I could begin asking questions and making doctor appointments. I went to the Internet. Recalling a speaker I heard at a conference a few years earlier discuss a prostate cancer support group known as Us TOO, I went online and found Us TOO, along with two other prostate cancer support groups. One was Malecare, a pre- and post-treatment program for gay men. Another group, sponsored by the American Cancer Society, was open to all men dealing with decisions about and outcomes of treatment regarding prostate cancer. After calls to each organization, I choose the group that had the most people in attendance and was closest to my home, Us TOO, and attended the next meeting. I also took my partner with me since I wanted to help him understand how this might impact both our lives. And the group did help him see choices I was facing and helped him try to imagine our future—as much as that was possible.

I went in to the group armed with the following two questions:

1. What expectations were you given by your physician going into your procedure?
2. What problems did you experience as a result of your medical procedure?

That was it, and I learned plenty.

The men in the group experienced a variety of outcomes from prostate cancer procedures. Some treatments had a negative impact on their bodies and their personal relationships, but the majority of the group overwhelmingly had positive outcomes. The negative or downside for some men involved not being told how to navigate their major medical insurance coverage from early- to late-stage cancer. The remainder of the comments largely surrounded the need for psychological comfort from caretakers pre- and post-treatment. I offer my observations of negative outcomes here, but have removed comments from individuals who were affected by expected complications associated with other medical conditions, such as people suffering from multiple illnesses simultaneously and those men who had complications associated with healing and their advanced age.

I asked the group, "So what surprised you about the outcome of your procedure?" One man who had had surgery said, "No one ever told me that my penis would shrink an inch." The room filled with laughter and signs of agreement. "Well, it often does as a result of the tissues retracting and scarring due to surgery. But it largely returns." Someone from across the room then shouted out, "It's true. But I was surprised when I began bleeding about six months out of surgery. It was very, very unusual and short-term, but it happened."

These twenty men seemed to experience very few post-treatment surprises. In addition, these comforting men also supplied me with information that proved invaluable in my decision-making process and future conversations with physicians. They quickly offered me the names of doctors, their specialty, length of procedural practice, along with their personality styles, staffing issues, and many times even their office phone numbers. One woman who was married to the man sitting with her suggested, "You know you can go to a radiologist or a surgeon, and then obtain a final collective opinion from an oncologist, if you want." That was exactly what I did. I also quickly learned how lucky I was to have had an early diagnosis via an annual PSA test, the support of a wonderful man, as well as the access to medical insurance. This was critical to the future success of my investigation.

One collection of comments from the group needs mentioning here, however. As stated earlier, the men in the group reported a need for psychological support. There were many, many complaints of medical staff not being supportive enough or in some cases not supportive at all. So then and there, I prepared myself for a degree of indifference to my condition.

That eventually proved to be helpful several times. I remember one particular instance of not being very fond of the physician who worked with me. He dropped into his chair, stared at me, and asked, "What can I do for you?" I thought, "Boy, he doesn't even pretend to modulate his voice." I reminded myself that we were not going to have a long-term relationship. I might see him six times in my life. Also, I reminded myself that he was trying to protect his emotions and focus on major surgical issue, while reducing personal prejudice and his treatment bias. And that was the reason for my visit.

I knew from teaching in a medical school that surgeons are known for not being very skilled in hand holding. So in our conversations I only expected him to explain the facts regarding my post-surgery plumbing: permanent erectile dysfunction remedied with Viagra or other erectile medication. I steered clear of personal matters unrelated to my health. I was open, however, by saying I was a gay man with a partner. I asked, "Will there be any issue regarding my partner's decision-making powers or his access to me?" No, he replied but I would need to see a social worker regarding some forms for emergency decisions.

From that point on, I went with the flow and asked the questions I had prepared:

What are the big studies and how do they relate to me (age, race, current medical condition, mental status, sexual orientation)?

How old was the study? I was looking for those conducted within the last three to five years.

How many people were involved in the study? The smaller the group, the less interested I was in the results.

What were the study results? The further out from the initial procedure, the more I trusted the outcomes.

What were the long-term effects identified by the studies? I needed to crosscheck each physician's knowledge of his area of specialization with that of other specialists.

What does the research say about the worst-case scenario? I needed to know how similar the study group members were to me and to determine mild, moderate, and severe negative outcomes.

How did the doctor select which patients he or she takes or doesn't take under his/her care? Physicians can select patients with only minimal needs. Therefore, their positive outcomes are usually high. So if the doctor was not selective in his patient population, I had a greater sense of confidence in his problem-solving abilities.

How often had the doctor performed this type of procedure in his lifetime?

When it comes to any invasive procedure, like surgery, what has been the infection rate of the doctor's patients? This is the most common form of complication and is tracked by hospitals, so physicians usually know the percent of post-op surgical infections.

What has been the doctor's success rate over time when it comes to side effects? Here your physician should also have some quantitative data to offer you on the physical side effects and resulting lifestyle changes over time.

After listening to answers to the above questions, I asked the doctor to compare what he knew of the newly developing robotic surgical techniques, which I was considering as an option. I had learned from an earlier meeting with the robotics surgeon that the procedure proposes to reduce in-hospital stays, infection rates, external scars, and improve nerve sparing when compared to traditional surgical methods.

He said, "Yeah, I know. I've done them. But I just don't get the point of it. If you place all of the small surgical scars together in a line, it's the same size as the traditional method. I mean I usually do it if the patient will lose time or pay from loss of work. It saves a few days. Other than that, I don't see the point."

So what's the research on it?

"There is some early research indicating that some patients are coming out with long-term urinary incontinence problems."

How many?

"It seems that about ten percent of the men have problems two years out of surgery. Interesting, but right now, we just don't know why."

Well, that's where the research would start then, wouldn't it?

"Yeah, that's true," he said, tilting his head in my direction.

And what do the nurses say when comparing care needed by patients who choose the robotic versus the traditional surgery?

"They say if you pull a sheet over the scars, you can't tell the difference between the two procedures."

I decided then to book my traditional surgery.

"Now?" he said with a surprise. "Really, you don't have to do it now. You can still look around."

"Yes, right now," I responded.

"Are you sure?" he asked again.

"Yup, let's follow the research outcomes."

Even though I had scheduled a surgery date, a week later I marched into an oncologist's office looking for a final opinion from a third party, just as the woman in the Us TOO support group had suggested. In the oncologist's opinion, radiology and surgery all offered equally good options. I then asked, "Which procedure would you say was the best option for you?" He said, "If it were me, I would want that thing out of me. And I would want it thrown in hazardous waste as soon as possible." I responded that every nurse and doctor I know personally had the same opinion.

I found that traditional surgical methods offered me the best treatment and physical outcome for predicting the highest survival potential. The research at the time for men around age fifty strongly favored surgical removal of the prostate. The majority of study results indicated that surgery offered reduced return cancer rates and prolonged life for the majority of patients. Surgery also offered me the option to use radiation in the future, should the cancer ever return. (Whereas, had I chosen radiation, I would not be eligible to use it again should the cancer return.) Hospital records suggest that there are no differences in patients' infections rates between those who selected robotic or traditional surgery. So the decision for me became clear. Again, my decision was based on the physician's experience as a surgeon, not just on comparisons of the procedures and their outcomes. These were only minimally discussed with the radiologist and surgeons.

I certainly had my moments of running to the hills with my fight-or-flight response to my illness. I remember thinking: "What about my partner and our sex life? What would it be like to never have the choice of children? How much pain would there be, and for how long?" One thing we know from the current brain research is the longer you wait to move on a stressful decision, the more the stress will increase.

In order to manage my worry demon, I took several communication-related steps. I talked about my cancer with only a few men I found in the Us TOO support group and with my partner, family, and friends whom I considered insightful. I avoided talking to dramatic personality types. This really reduced my worry time and increased my decision-making abilities.

In addition, I helped reduce my stress level and cleared my thinking with meditation techniques. I did them twice a day for approximately fifteen minutes.

The process involves the following:

1. Sit comfortably in a quiet place with your spine straight.
2. Allow your breathing to flow and catch the changing rhythms of your in- and out-breath.
3. Notice your attention wandering off to memories,

feelings, and thoughts, which will happen often.

4. Label each memory, feeling, or thought as you come to recognize it.

5. Gently bring your awareness back to your breathing, which is your focal point.

6. Remain curious about "watching" your memories, feelings, and thoughts as they come and go without judgment.

My aim was not to arrive anywhere, but to be fully in the present moment, one after another, aware only of my breath. This simple technique, done twice a day, really did help me move away from worry, which also helped me make better decisions related to my cancer. In addition, this meditative process also aided me through difficult conversations with minimally supportive people, who were associated with insurance issues and medical care.

I chose traditional surgery like most of the gay men in the Malecare cancer support group who had partners; men in that group who did not have partners tended to opt for radiation or watchful waiting as their treatment option. As for my post-surgical outcomes, I have lived with them for over three years now. I miss the strength of former orgasms and my sperm. My partner was wonderful and overwhelmingly supportive, never complaining. But life and our relationship have changed. Urinary incontinence during sex was an issue of embarrassment for me and repulsive to him. He would suddenly jump up during sex, be still, and freeze. Then he would look at me, and I would know. I must have had some urine leakage. I felt sad and sorry for both of us. So I learned to adjust my water intake and timed my meditations for sustaining my erections. I miss the casual and spontaneous attitude of my youth. But I miss many things about my youthful body. The truth is I am in an aging body, and I have adapted. Sex is still possible, though more calculated on my part. I live with the surgical outcomes and think I made the right decision for me.

My decision was based on investigating how doctors think, not just the pluses and minuses of different medical procedures. Finally, I will conclude my own unscientific observations by saying I have noticed that about ten percent of the men in the support groups I have attended who have long term urinary problems are also the men who have undergone robotic surgical procedure. But perhaps this is just a sampling problem on my part. Future research will have to give us that answer.

Personal Issues to Consider Before and After Radical Prostatectomy

Milton Sonday

The aim of this essay is to recount my own experiences as a gay man dealing with prostate cancer (PCa) from diagnosis through prostatectomy and recovery, and to share what I experienced in the hope that other men will benefit from what I have learned. I should say at the start that, for reasons I cannot explain, at no point in the medical process was I overly alarmed or frightened by the prospect of surgery.

Many of the points that I raise are not limited to gay men, but being gay made it relatively easy for me to discuss sexual issues that are irrevocably associated with prostate cancer. Straight men would very likely find it difficult to have such talks with their doctors, therapists, other men, and women. It seems to me that it is a not well-hidden secret that many women are as interested in male sexuality as gay men, but I doubt that this holds true for straight men. Therefore, I feel that gay men have a responsibility to speak out about prostate cancer in general and about the changes in sexual perceptions and performance that prostate cancer treatment might impose in particular.

Do not be surprised if your doctors do not volunteer very much information; this seems to be the norm, provided that the basics are covered. The latter should include the virulence of the cancer expressed as the Gleason score, the benefits and drawbacks of all treatments (with perhaps a bias in the direction of their specialty or favored treatment modality), the potential effects of various treatments on your sexual performance and/or urinary functioning, as well as some information about support groups and literature. It is difficult to draw the line between basic information and too much information; for example, there were certain facts that I did not want to know, such as the exact location and length of the incision and the possible complications, because I knew they would scare me. I was not about to worry about complications that in any case would have to be dealt with later. The issues that did alarm me during my recovery were personal, and various health care providers could have discussed them with me, but they did not, and it is these issues that I will point out later in this essay.

It is imperative that you trust your general practitioner (GP) and urologist/surgeon. If you don't, find another. It would be extremely helpful if your trusted GP has had successful prostate surgery himself, as mine had. It was because of his diligent testing that my cancer was detected. My GP is also gay and, given his personal experience, I felt his own urologist/surgeon, who is not gay, came well-recommended.

My cancer was detected as a result of steadily rising PSA numbers. While a PSA count is not in itself an indication of cancer, it is known that cancer cells generally produce much more PSA than normal cells; however, counts may be way above average for many men who are cancer free. My PSA count had been going up gradually for a number years and warranted five biopsies starting in 2000. I became increasingly anxious because my dad had had prostate cancer, although at a more advanced age, and he ultimately died of congenital heart disease. I was sixty-six. My diagnosis in March 2006 came as a sort of relief. No more waiting for what I felt was inevitable. I was immediately prepared to follow through with treatment. When my cancer was diagnosed, my PSA count was 20, and its virulence was rated at a Gleason score of 6 (3 +3) on an ascending scale from 2 to 10.

My urologist/surgeon essentially presented me with only one treatment option: a radical prostatectomy, or surgical removal of my prostate. He did not recommend radiation as a primary treatment because it hardens tissues and makes subsequent surgery more invasive and difficult. Radiation would be an option if follow-up treatment became necessary after surgery. Whether or not my cancer might have been delayed by drinking tomato juice with a few drops of oil of oregano and taking Saw Palmetto (see glossary), I have no idea. Whether or not my cancer might have been reversed by alternative homeopathic means, I do not know. These regimens require strong faith, of which I have very little. I requested surgery as soon as possible, and it was scheduled for mid-April 2006. In retrospect, I was glad that I did not need to explore treatment options and thereby learn about possible complications; which is not to say I was not apprehensive. I became alarmed months after my surgery when I read about prejudice against gay men and ignorance or avoidance of gay issues. I felt overwhelmed trying to absorb the pros and cons of the basic treatment options: active surveillance (wait and see); prostatectomy (radical surgery with incision or laproscopic surgery with fiber optic instruments); radiation therapy (burning); cryotherapy (freezing), or hormone therapy (chemical castration). I realized that prior to surgery I could not have coped with very much of this information. I thought of surgery as a professional procedure that was to be performed by a knowledgeable and well-trained team, and that is what I experienced.

After you receive a diagnosis of PCa, you need to be prepared to take care of yourself, even if you have a partner/spouse and good friends. Be able to put your arms around yourself and give yourself a huge hug. Find a role model for self-care. Mine was my mother, who was a registered nurse and whose care and attention to her patients were thoroughly professional. She dealt with medical emergencies and treatments head-on and she was thoroughly focused on her role as a caretaker. In other words, it was "business as usual," just as it became for me when I was confronted with major surgery for the first time in my life.

In spite of the fact that prostate surgery is characterized by the medical profession as "improved," "commonplace," and "highly effective," there is no escaping the fact that it is major surgery. Do not let this alarm you. Develop your self-care system and try not to panic. If possible, schedule your surgery for late spring or early fall. Good weather will encourage you to walk very soon after surgery and you will feel more comfortable in your home.

Many issues and procedures that arise as a result of having prostate cancer require your full attention and can be emotionally draining, so look for and savor the humane, humorous, and bizarre moments. I found it very helpful to record these experiences in a diary.

Prior to Surgery

Go to the hospital a few days before pre-surgery tests. Locate the elevator to the floor on which the surgery will be done and other appropriate offices; then there will be no need to panic about the exact location of the hospital and how long it takes to get there.

Stock your refrigerator, freezer, and cupboard with enough easy-to-prepare foods for about three days. You will be encouraged to walk about two days after surgery, or sooner while you are in the hospital. I was in the hospital for three and a half days. Walks to the supermarket after you leave the hospital can be beneficial. Take along a friend to carry heavy stuff or have the supermarket deliver. The canned baked beans a friend recommended never tasted so good.

Buy several pairs of loose-fitting pants (a size too large is ideal). You will need diapers. Get a package in advance and try one on. Treat this as a fun dress-up experience. Pretend you are having a Halloween party and invite a friend or your lover/spouse to join you.

When you wake up in the recovery room, you will have been outfitted with a catheter inserted in your penis. Do not let this alarm you. Find out in advance of surgery what a catheter is and does. A catheter is inconvenient, but it is actually useful. Urine is collected in a pouch that, for obvious reasons, must be kept lower than your penis. The pouch is flat and expands as it is filled and it can be strapped to your thigh or hung next to your bed. Rig up a way to hang the bag at the side of your bed. I attached a C-clamp to my bedside table that functioned as a hook. Hospital staff will show you how to strap the bag to your thigh and drain it. There will be an elastic strap at the top and bottom of the pouch that you will wrap around your thigh. I hope you are told, and if not, remember to turn the pouch under at the bottom. Apply baby powder to your thigh where the straps touch your skin to avoid irritation; get this in advance if you do not already have it in your medicine cabinet.

The most alarming thing about the catheter is that your bladder will reject it because it does not tolerate the irritation caused by the catheter and the balloon that holds in place. I was not warned about rejection-spasms in advance nor did I read about them in advance, and I panicked when I realized that urine was leaking out at the tip of my penis; it felt as if the catheter had come out, but that was not the case. The sensation is very uncomfortable but not painful. Unfortunately, spasms do not let up until the catheter is removed, so take deep breaths and relax when they occur. You should be given an antibacterial gel to apply to the tip of your penis while you are outfitted with the tube. Have a generous supply of towels available to soak up leaked urine or get a plastic-lined pad made for the mattress of a child's crib. I coped with my catheter for two weeks; this provided ample time for the incision around the urethra at the base of the bladder to heal.

Prior to surgery, my urologist/surgeon recommended the Kegel exercise. These exercises consist of a rhythmic tightening and relaxing of the circular muscle fibers at the neck of the bladder and the sphincter muscles beneath the bladder surrounding the urethra that, which when tightened, help stop the flow of urine. These exercises may well have helped me regain full continence and had an unanticipated benefit that I will point out later.

Pack for the hospital as if you are going to a nudist colony; you will be outfitted with hospital clothing. Leave your jewelry at home. Remember to take important phone numbers.

Ask a friend or your lover/spouse to be your advocate during your stay in the hospital and ask him or her to find out when you are to be released and if you can walk out the front door. If the hospital insists on a wheelchair, try not to be embarrassed; enjoy the ride. In any case, you cannot leave the hospital alone. I would recommend a car service and not a taxicab. The cab driver my advocate and I hailed insisted on competitive driving and I had to elevate myself on straight arms to avoid bouncing on the seat. Have your advocate bring you an inflatable doughnut-shaped cushion. While sitting was not too uncomfortable, I used mine at home and took it with me to the opera, along with my external plumbing system; the experience was a hoot.

While in the Hospital

There is so much going on around you in the hospital that you will have no time to think, let alone have the ability to think clearly. Unrelenting activity made it impossible for me to get a full night's sleep. The Xanax I asked for was minimally effective. My short stay in the hospital demanded my full attention and I could not have coped with many visitors, so do not be shy about telling friends or family not to visit. Mobility is limited and there is no privacy; nor did it help that I was one of four in the room.

Do not hesitate to walk as soon as you are told to do so. It may seem awkward at first to walk with the wheeled IV stand holding your urine and other IV fluid bags so do it with flair. I experienced no pain and found it a great relief to be on my own and mobile.

Early on, you will be asked if you passed gas, and after being asked many times you will begin to feel anxious if you have not. There is also the annoying wait for your first bowel movement, and I did not have mine until soon after I was released from the hospital. Be sure to have a home supply of a stool softener. For some reason, I was not able to read or watch TV with full comprehension or concentrate on music for the next two weeks. These otherwise normal distractions were replaced by the pleasure and pride I felt in taking care of myself.

My GP suggested I hire private duty nurses, which sounded like a good idea, so I did. It turned out to be not worth the expense. The two private nurses in consecutive shifts were clearly not liked by the regular staff and their care lacked the finesse of the excellent nurses and aides on duty. Nevertheless, it can be a reasonable option.

I was warned in advance that hospital food would be terrible, but just how terrible was shocking. My two private nurses were essentially not allowed to leave my bedside, which I found quite annoying; nonetheless I could not have trusted them to bring me something tolerable to eat. Put a good friend or your lover/spouse on alert for a food delivery as soon as you are allowed to have solid food, which will probably not be possible until your last day in the hospital in any case, so there is no urgency.

At Home Alone: The First Few Days

Don't be alarmed if you panic soon after returning to your home. As soon as my caretaker got me home and helped me with a bit of food shopping and went on his way, I began to shiver, my heart started pounding, and I burst out crying. It was then that the shock of what I had just experienced and was about to face hit me with full force. My panic remained high for most of the day and with less intense force over the next few days. This was the most surprising event of my recovery; one that I was never warned about, which became the primary motivating force for me to share my experiences here. At the time, it never occurred to me to request anti-depression medication. For the next two weeks, all I could think about was caring for myself; the rest of the world was blocked out. On some level this was one of the most purely personal, even peaceful, times of my life; another was when my partner died nineteen years ago. There were no distractions from the outside world, partly by choice, except for a few close friends, some of whom joined me for walks in the park. In a very short time I began feeling my mind and body joyfully pulling itself together and healing day-by-day. Fortunately, I enjoy cooking for myself and that was a major factor in my gradually improving both physically and emotionally. The outside world eventually forced its way in, but ever since I have tried to keep a section of my mind clear for myself, something that I previously found difficult to achieve. Eventually I had a bowel movement, and who would have thought that it would be a significant event and one that I would write about?

The Process of Recovery

There is probably no clear answer to the question of how long it takes to recover. The effect of anesthesia lasts a long time, but its effects are subtle and difficult to recognize and can be confused with effects we associate with aging, such as difficulty remembering names and what was or was not in the refrigerator.

Pain Management

I was never anxious about pain, but I was relieved to see posters suggesting management consultation in the pre-surgery testing area in the hospital. It turned out that prior to my surgery I was invited to join a study of the use of a beta-blocker to reduce pain. At no point after my surgery was I in pain, and I was amused to discover that pain, aside from levels of tolerance, has various definitions or interpretations. When the representatives of the study asked if I was in pain, I did not know how to answer because I assumed they meant, "Did I feel something sharp or stabbing?" What they actually expected me to describe was a sensation that I could only characterize as an uncomfortable ache, as if my bowels were tightly blocked, which in fact they were.

The Catheter

Removing the catheter is painless and after it is removed you may indeed miss it because you will experience incontinence, or the inability to stop the flow of urine; hence the use of diapers—they really work. Chances are that you will regain continence, but how long that will take varies considerably from man to man, and some men do not. At some point you will hopefully be able to stop wearing a diaper and start to use a "guard" that is designed to adhere to your underwear; it is like having a codpiece and will dramatically fill out your cloth-covered crotch. Take your leftover, unused diapers to a care facility for elderly men. One of the benefits of surgery, other than the obvious elimination of cancer, is that your flow of urine will typically be smooth and strong, just as it was when you were a kid and challenged in long distance pissing contests. Bowel movements also improve.

Your Real Friends

If you are a very private person who takes care of himself and is not a complainer, you probably did not tell too many people about your cancer and surgery. Review those you did and did not tell. If there were some among those you did tell who did not respond or avoided your issue, consider what that says about them and how to handle it. Ask yourself why you chose not to tell some people. Do not feel guilty about not telling them and offer an honest explanation if challenged. A housecleaning of your address book and guest list may be in order.

During my recovery I was not in a relationship. This may have been a positive factor in my case because it freed me to focus my caretaking on myself and not direct it to another man, who may or may not have been able to cope with the challenge. Being single allowed me to choose the people with whom I felt comfortable to ask to run errands for me and/or visit with me.

Getting on With Your Sex Life

Because sex as uninhibited pleasure is very much a part of gay male identity, it is essential to learn how your sexual apparatus and system works. In The Joy of Gay Sex, the authors observe, "few activities involve so many different parts and structures of the body as sex does." They start their discussion of sex by suggesting that the primary sex organ is not your cock, but your brain; the latter is characterized as a circuit breaker. They go on to say that three elements determine how our brain affects sexuality:

genetics, which determine sexual orientation; molding by social structure; and finally, personal and specific experiences. Masters and Johnson (1966) state that there are four stages in a male's sexual response: excitement; the plateau reached in an advanced state of arousal; orgasm, which includes ejaculatory inevitability to the point of no return; and resolution, which is the return of the body to its normal state. The authors go on to discuss our double nervous system: There is the central nervous system for voluntary movements such as with skeletal muscles and those that affect audio and visual stimulation; and there is the autonomic nervous system for involuntary responses of internal organs such as breathing and maintaining body temperature and the responses in our genitals. The autonomic nervous system has two subsystems, one that speeds up the heart rate (sympathetic) and another that slows down the heart rate (parasympathetic); both interact with erections.

Obviously, the biological function of male sex is to impregnate a female so that sperm fertilizes an egg that develops into a fetus. Sperm travels from both testicles, where it is made, through tiny tubes called the vas deferens to the upper ends of the seminal vesicles, two glands at the base of the bladder. It is here that fructose, a sugar to nourish the sperm, is added, as well as an enzyme that clumps into globs that we know can stick to your belly after you come.

The function of the walnut-sized prostate gland, located just below the urinary bladder that surrounds the urethra (the tube that leads from the bladder through the prostate, past the urinary sphincter, and out the penis ending in a slit through which urine and seminal fluid pass), is to produce enzymes that liquefy the mass holding the semen. During sexual stimulation, semen collects in the ejaculatory ducts where the vas deferens from both testicles Join the seminal vessels and mixes with secretions of the prostate.

The secretions of the prostate comprise about a third of the ejaculate, giving it its whitish color.

Erection begins with sensory and mental stimulation and occurs when blood fills two cylindrical chambers that run the length of the penis parallel to the urethra. These two cylinders of spongy tissue surrounded by a tough fibrous covering fill most of the penis. In a healthy male, the tissues become engorged with blood during sexual excitement, causing the penis to expand. As the spongy tissues fill with blood, they push against the fibrous sheath, making the penis hard.

What is known as pre-cum is a fluid produced by the pea-sized Cowper's gland that functions separately from the prostate. The scrotum and testes undergo some interesting changes during sex. The skin of the scrotal sac thickens and contracts, while the testes increase in size because of the engorgement of blood. The testes are also pulled up within the sac until they press against the wall of the pelvis. This elevation of the testes anticipates ejaculation and is necessary for it to occur.

When a climax is reached, a spinal reflex causes contractions to the muscles in the penis, urethra, and the prostate, thereby pouring their contents into the urethra to be propelled or ejaculated out through the tip of the penis. Contractions are the beginning of ejaculation and nothing can stop it once the point of inevitability is reached. Ejaculation is a total body response involving a complex series of minute actions; and is not a shame that a gland the size of an ordinary walnut can cause devastating havoc for what is set up to be a hugely pleasurable experience. Ejaculation is the physical part, the propulsion of seminal fluid or cum. Orgasm is the peak feeling in sex that in men usually occurs during ejaculation, but not always.

Sexual Dysfunction

Removing the prostate eliminates the possibility of an ejaculation, but there is an orgasm. Sperm that is produced is absorbed into the testes. When the surgeon removes a man's prostate, the muscle that closes his bladder allowing his ejaculate to move out of his penis rather than back into his bladder is destroyed. While still perfectly capable of experiencing an orgasm, no ejaculate comes out. This will not be the sort of orgasm that you are familiar with, but one that seems to grow and be contained deeper within you. An orgasm takes place in the brain and is not eliminated by loss of the prostate. This brings us back to the important role of the nervous system in sex and emphasizes the need to relax before trying to achieve an orgasm with or without an erection. For many of us this requires a bit of adjustment, so evoke the components of romance. Fortunately, a radical prostatectomy does not affect the anus or rectum. Reduced ability to achieve an erection and maintain it is certainly frustrating and at times may make us feel hopeless. My doctors as well as my psychotherapist insisted that I not ignore this issue. Remember to ask your surgeon whether his procedure is nerve-sparing. After surgery, ask the surgeon if some or all of the nerve bundles on each side of the prostate were spared. These bundles of nerves play a crucial role in the retrieval of your erection. Even if the nerve bundles are not removed during radical prostatectomy, they may still sustain damage and are very slow to heal. However, even if the bundles are not injured during surgery, some men will experience erectile dysfunction afterward; the reasons are unclear. Another common reason for difficulty with erections is that the veins of the penis may have suffered trauma during surgery and are unable to keep blood trapped inside the penis.

About four months after surgery, I began to deal seriously with erectile dysfunction. I became aware of varying satisfactory degrees to which my penis could and would be filled with blood while not becoming fully erect. It was not necessary to be fully erect to play with my cock and enjoy a blowjob or have my playmate enjoy what he was doing.

My plumbing system confused urination with blood swelling in the penis. Finding the pleasure and bits of humor in this became a challenge, so I stood over the toilet or bath tub, gathered together used towels and kept them close at hand, or, as my patient friend/playmate suggested, protected my sofa and bed with a plastic-lined crib mattress cover. The urge to urinate and the sensation in the tip of my penis made me feel like I needed to urinate, but the sensations were unpleasant. Blood swelling the penis at some point begins to override urination, so don't give up. While I do not think of myself as being particularly prudish, a frank discussion with my straight urologist about an erection was in order and I approached it with some apprehension. Imagine being in a sterile, brightly illuminated examination room with the urologist who guides you through the process of inserting a thin rod containing the magic potion into your penis and who has to show you himself how to complete the process and then leaves you to rub your member for fifteen minutes before he returns to check on the results. Results were positive and my only option after the doctor completed his paperwork and left the room was to put on my pants, zip up, walk out of the office, and enter the subway with a silly grin on my face. The inserted medicine, Alprostadil, left me feeling swelled and a bit achy, but not unpleasantly so, and as far as I am concerned is a much better option than injecting a drug into my penis using a needle, although this has been described to me as a simple and painless procedure using Caverject.

Unfortunately, the insurance system is extremely parsimonious about reimbursing erection-enhancing products. This is yet another result of living in a culture that denies that it encourages sex for pleasure. One way around this is to pay full-price and wait out the required amount of time between refills of a prescription.

A cheaper way to get blood to flow into the penis is to use a vacuum pump, but this has limited application and I have been warned that using it can damage blood vessels.

Sexual Pleasure

In order for an erection to occur, a whole constellation of things needs to be in alignment. Your nervous and vascular systems have to be capable of responding properly, and your emotions have to be capable of aiding or at least not impeding the process. Anything, physical or emotional, that gets in the way of sufficient blood getting into and staying in the penis can cause problems. Many prescription drugs, not to mention alcohol, tobacco, and street drugs may impede erections

I don't know if I was ever compulsive about sex; I enjoyed it and certainly took my never-failing erection for granted. Now that I have had a radical prostatectomy, I think a lot about sex and warn myself that I must not become obsessive. Obsession is not a good attitude for me. I am being pro-active in working towards an improved erection. I can no longer take my erection for granted and it takes some effort and a lot of energy to achieve it. I am reminded that, prior to diagnosis, my GP routinely suggested I jerk off three times a week, and now I am told to attempt an erection every day. I guess practice makes perfect. Nevertheless, a penis, like the rest of the body, goes through a life cycle and, for men who have had a prostatectomy at a time when reactions are not as hard and ejaculation is less powerful, longer recovery time is required.

Whether or not my cock will become stiff enough for

fucking is not all that important to me; a cock must be stiffer for anal penetration than for vaginal. In its place is increased pleasure in sensual touching and being touched. Ejaculation is no longer a goal, and I am reminded that there are some positive references for what is known as a dry orgasm, such as certain Buddhist sects that avoid ejaculation and the objectives of Body Electric, a group of men who gather for non-orgasmic encounters. There is no point in looking back with regret.

The new combination of the familiar and now subtly changed sensations may indeed be more pleasurable, but this is tinged with regret for the loss of full sexual performance and youth. My sexual sensations are different, notably increased tingling of the tip of my penis as a climax is built and achieved.

Your reaction to gay sexual stereotypes may change as did mine. The image of a huge engorged cock and a long arch of ejaculated semen, which was never my favorite image anyway, now appeal to me even less. Men no longer have the same erotic appeal. More specifically, I am less anxious about approaching and talking to gay men that I find attractive and less likely to second-guess how I might perform. Actually, I am looking at attractive men more now than in the past. I seem to be less shy. Eroticism is now based more on imagined and actual sensual touching, stroking, and holding; far less on super-active participation in fucking, sucking, and so on. Some of this is built into the aging process that includes reduced libido, so those of us who have been forced to adjust to new definitions of sexual involvement are in a good position to advise older men who have not had such an abrupt change yet face similar challenges (Harris, 2005).

Penises do not have to be hard to produce pleasure. A soft penis has just as many nerve endings as a hard one and is therefore capable of generating good feelings. Whether it is exactly as enjoyable as an erect penis is difficult to say.

Although the number of nerve endings doesn't change, it is possible that the engorgement of the hard penis with blood amplifies the sensations. Some men say it is more pleasurable to be stimulated with an erection, and some say it does not make any difference. And it is also possible to have an orgasm with a soft penis.

This is your opportunity to try out various cock rings, nipple clamps, and other stimulation toys that suit your fancy. Remember that sex is meant to be pleasurable. Do not give up on erotic fetishes and images: cocks, asses, nipples, the curve of a well-formed chest, the curving in of the lower spine. So disconnect the phone, turn off the computer, dim the lamps, light a candle, take a bath, or as Napoleon supposedly wrote to Josephine, "Don't bathe, I will be home in a month." Play your favorite romantic music, watch a hot porn video, play with your toys, enjoy your body, and have a ball. If you can do it with another man, so much the better. Now I understand why an attractive and sensual man I met several years ago created an altar to a self-created gay sex god with a large assortment of toys and images of sexy men. You never know when what seems bizarre in another man might someday become acceptable and meaningful to you.

I was pleased to learn that my post-surgery libido was not dead. Prior to the detection of cancer, I rekindled my interest in drawing and joined a workshop that focuses on erotic male nudes. While drawing, your libido is put on hold, but there is no denying that at some point the urge to jerk off cries out to be satisfied.

My sexual confidence returned slowly and, not having a lover/spouse, I was fortunate to have a very understanding friend who joined me in exploring a wide array of sensual and sexual pleasures. At first I was shy about showing my body and revealing my scar, as well a bulged section of my gut pushed aside by the thick line caused by the stapled-together incision, but with his help, I gradually overcame this inhibition. I did not apply Vitamin E to my scar as Carmela Soprano did to Tony's scar on the TV show The Sopranos.

No doubt there are probably guys who like scars.

Much of the pleasure of anal intercourse is the repeated rubbing and pounding of the prostate, and without a prostate, you must rely on other sensations. Enter the Kegel exercises. If you do them conscientiously, you may notice that the strengthened sphincter muscle that closes the anus increases or enhances the pleasure of anal intercourse. Most gay men already know this, but if you thought that you would never be fucked again, controlled use of this magic muscle is a way to keep in rhythmic contact with your partner and provide him with an added dose of pleasure. Perhaps I should have done the Kegel exercises with a dildo.

In addition to dealing with impotence and erectile dysfunction, there will be follow-up visits with your urologist/surgeon.

Conclusion

At some point while I was patching together the components of a man's sexual system, it occurred to me that removal of the prostate gland and possibly other treatments as well, amounts to sterilization. Removing the prostate necessitates the severing of the vas deferens—in other words, a vasectomy. This realization may be yet another blow to a man's psyche, but one that should not be dwelt upon at great length.

I was out as a gay man both personally and professionally for decades, and I did not experience gay-related fears or anxieties when forced to deal with prostate cancer. I did not think my cancer had anything to do with being gay nor did having it significantly diminish my self-worth and self-image. I grieved for myself and went through a brief period of mourning, but not as severely or as prolonged as what I experienced following the death of my lover/spouse who died of AIDS in the mid-1980s. Both experiences—Terry's death and my cancer—gave renewed meaning to my life, a sensation that is as valuable now as it was then, but more so now as I realize that I am entering the next age cycle of my life.

Some men prefer to learn about treatment options and their potential side effects before they make a treatment decision. If you are one of them I suggest that you address questions to your doctors, join a support group, participate in dialogues via the Internet, and consult the books that are referenced at the end of this volume.

Suggestions for Those Considering Invasive Procedures

"Paul Jarod"

A jump in my PSA score told me it was time to be proactive; it had been escalating and now was up nearly a full point in a year, rising from 3.0 to 3.9. My primary care physician was laidback about it all. He said, "You can wait and see or get an insurance referral for a prostate biopsy." The referral made most sense to me.

The urologist for the biopsy was already a known entity a doctor I had seen for testicular pain a few years prior. Back then he had explained that I had something fairly common, a benign epididymal cyst, and that he himself had one in his left sac. This eased my concern. While still in professional bounds, it felt more like two guys talking about everyday ball pain than a weighty clinical conversation.

Throughout the biopsy, my urologist was a strong communicator volunteering what he was doing step-by-step and giving me signals as to when to expect the various probe insertions. This was a welcome contrast to cold, assembly-line urologists that I had encountered in prior years.

The PSA results were not definitive. There was cancer, but in a small portion of the biopsy samples taken. The Gleason score was 6 (3+3). At age sixty-two, I might outlive the threat of the malignancy there, but then again, maybe not. There was no way to be sure. Again, the urologist gave me just the right balance of science and conversation in explaining my biopsy results. Importantly, he armed me with a book about prostate cancer before I left his office. This 300-plus-page book was mine to keep. It laid out all the major options and answered many of my questions and concerns. The doctor had also given me his assurance that no immediate decision was needed given my circumstances; even if I chose a treatment, I could not begin it for at least six weeks, since the body needs to heal after the biopsy.

After reading the book and doing some Internet searches, I decided to take a vacation that had already been on the calendar. While away I would weigh the options with a minimal amount of anxiety. The doctor's talk and the background reading had helped me to focus rather than to panic.

I found the decision process of what to do surprisingly individual. Each man selects the approach that seems to fit him best when he weighs the pros and cons. By doing this there is some sense of control, some feeling of empowerment regarding how to proceed. This can be quite helpful when there is a threat to the male equipment that tends to be pre-wired in our brains as our source of power and potency.

After my trip, I told the urologist that I wanted to have open surgery (a radical prostatectomy). It may be a more invasive approach than some other procedures, but I was after two possible end benefits. First, it gives the surgeon greater potential to physically detect affected tissue during surgery and to decide whether or not to spare the nerves according to what seems best for overall health and ultimate survival. Second, it allows the future option of radiation therapy, if ever needed, should some malignant tissue linger. I learned that it is much more difficult to do the reverse since having surgery after radiation is much trickier and a less recommended course of action.

My urologist had a couple of notable surgeons for me to consider, and the one I selected turned out to be just as personable and communicative as my urologist. This was a valuable extra once I was sure of his technical skills. Overall, my surgery went well and my routine blood work results continue to be encouraging.

Issues to Consider Before and After Surgery

Although I felt I was in very good hands with the physician and the hospital, there were things I wish I had known ahead of time. Even in the best of situations, every detail cannot be communicated; and even if communicated, there is so much to process that not all of it stays in the memory bank; not to mention that anxiety gets in the way of absorbing new material.

Things I Would Liked to Have Known or Had Underscored Before Surgery

1. You may need to hound the office to get your biopsy routed to the next doctor in time. Knowing how busy my urologist's office can be I kept calling to see if the assistant would pass along my biopsy results for my first appointment with the surgeon. It was good that I kept on top of things because it just sat there until the surgeon's own assistant got involved and moved the process along. What I did not realize is that the surgeon himself needed a few days to have an independent lab look at the glass slides and give a professional second opinion. Others have told me they had similar timing snags with biopsy "pass-alongs." I would advise one to check and re-check that the biopsy results are sent out from the first office as well as received at the second.

2. When it comes to the surgeon's success record, you may have to depend on what he/she tells you. Surprisingly, it may only be the surgeon who has the statistics of how many procedures he has done and what the success-rate details are. With this you have to decide if you can trust the

track record that the surgeon is telling you about. Meanwhile, there are some other peripheral aspects that you may be able to check online as I did: Is the surgeon board-certified? Have any charges been filed against the doctor? Has the doctor lost any hospital privileges due to practice issues? Naturally, it is also helpful to get word-of-mouth impressions about the doctor through personal networking when possible.

3. The hospital food may not do the trick for your digestion. The books all impress upon you to keep your digestive system regular after surgery; that you may not even be released from the hospital until you can move your bowels. The menus at my hospital did not provide anything to help with this; there were far too many binding starches, no fruit, and very few liquids. So I went to Plan B and had friends bring me fruit, prunes, and so forth. That is the only way I was able to get the pipes working again.

4. Get up and stretch while you can to ease bloating discomfort. My one regret at the hospital was not asking to get up before bedtime on the second night after surgery. During the whole stay, the only problem I had was from bloating, and by the time I was experiencing it, the night nurse said she could not let me get up and assist me walking because the late shift was understaffed. I lay awake all night, just waiting to be able to get up and stretch for the much-needed relief from the gas bloating.

5. Have a helping hand at home. Once home from the hospital, compromised stomach muscles may prevent some simple tasks you never gave a second thought to. I was able to walk and do everyday chores, but getting up on my own was another story after open surgery. It is critical to pre-plan to have someone in your household for the first two or three days if only to give you a pull up from the chair or bed and to help getting those socks on. Once I got up from the bed or a chair, I was fine, but having a buddy's arm to lean on was essential for me until my third day at home.

6. Move that bed ahead of time. If your bed is against the wall, think about moving it out a bit before you go to the hospital so that there is room for the night catheter bag when you get home. In the same way, think in advance about things you might want out of the back of the closet or from the top shelf of the cupboards; it is not easy to reach or stretch very far while you are healing.

Things I Would Have Liked to Have Known After Surgery

1. Doctors may simply want to know about "non-cloudy urine." When the doctor or nurse would ask me by phone if the catheter bag urine was clear yet, I was unnecessarily alarmed, thinking that my urine needed to be free of that pink tinge (some blood in the urine). All that the medical people were actually concerned with was if the urine was cloudy or clear; tint was something secondary.

2. Swollen man-parts may be included. After an internal operation north of my pubes, I was very surprised to see that my ball sacs and penis looked vacuum-pumped. Not that I minded the swelling (no pain involved), but I was quite concerned about the black-and-blue coloration (maroon-and-blue actually). I was told this discoloration can be a natural part of the healing until swelling goes down, so then I was able to rest easier as it gradually returned to normal over a few weeks time.

3. How far is that daily walk supposed to be? Several of the source books I read recommended walks for facilitating healing and suggested increasing the distance a little each day. I took the textbook advice, but did not know how much to extend the walking increments. I eventually calculated that even my early walks worked out to be about two miles; probably more than the doctor intended. In hindsight I should have asked the doctor just how long a walk to take each day.

4. Urine leakage is often an unsteady progression toward control. The progress with urinary continence can be unpredictable. I expected it would be an upward climb but found my continence progressed in stops, starts, and backsliding. Improvement can be so gradual and dragged out that it can be a real surprise to wake up one day and find you can get by wearing regular briefs and no absorption pads.

5. Prostate removal is no guarantee of powerhouse whizzing. The one thing I thought prostate surgery would deliver was better peeing. I thought for sure there would be a quicker stream when stepping up to the urinal, stronger streams overall, and also fewer nighttime trips to the bathroom. But this is apparently not true for all patients. My system is "normal" but I sometimes still stand and wait at the urinal instead of peeing like the racehorse I had hoped I would be. I still get up for bathroom breaks two or three times a night. My doctor said that it might just be an embedded habit from pre-surgery years.

6. Silicone sheeting can help with scarring. Scars are said to take six months to a year to heal as the pink fades. The latest literature recommends simply using silicone on the scar for healing. This is often in the form of clear silicone that sticks like a bandage or alternately a type that rubs on in a silicone cream form. I found the silicone very soothing and believe it does work to reduce the scarring.

Sexual Tips to Consider Post-Surgery

Although each man is wired differently and has to find or rediscover his own sensuality at his own pace, I found several things worked for me as I began to reclaim my sexuality and sensuality.

1. Standing up may help you get it up better. Several guys I have talked to agree that, before surgery, our penises were most likely to get hard relaxing in bed; automatically

stiffening nightly for a JO in the sack, having dream state erections, and waking up with a rigid piss hard-on. How I wish I had those now! But to our surprise, after surgery, the most relaxed sitting or reclining position does nothing for arousal. I have been getting more aroused when on my feet. Yet the minute I try to sit down, I lose whatever sexual tension I have built up, even if there is a hot DVD on. The bottom line is that some of us guys have to fight the urge to lie back if we want to get some response.

2. A randy day can be a wet day. Even after I was able to toss away the urine absorption pads, I found that on days when my libido was in full force, I would often shoot off urine like a trigger-happy water pistol. So I learned to have some toweling and a thick bathmat ready to throw down in front of my penis path. If you are getting frisky with a buddy or even giving yourself a hand-job, you never know when you are going to squirt some urine, so be prepared. It simply feels like the pipes are open for cum/pre-cum so the urine seems to take a free ride down the penile chute.

3. The shower is a very fitting JO location. When I got the OK from the doctor to masturbate again (a few weeks after the catheter was removed) I found the shower was a good place to give myself a morning yank. The research is showing we need to stimulate the nerves and spongy tissues, upholding the old saying, "use it or lose it." The shower is such an ideal place for this because you are standing up, which can help toward an erection. The warm water stimulates blood flow, and the tub is certainly a better alternative for an unscheduled pee-squirt than the living room carpet.

4. And while you are in that shower, get creative, explore! Pay attention to your erogenous zones. We are not just wired to our dicks alone. After surgery I wanted to spend more time on these erogenous zones, like the nipples, particularly when I could not depend on a stiff erection. Even though I had not been into water sports prior to

surgery, I found the sensation of that unexpected orgasmic pee-shoot to be an erotic charge along my shaft. And who knows what other things I might discover over time.

5. When to attempt anal sex. If it is difficult to ask the doctor directly when it is safe to engage in back-door sexual activity, consider what I did. I asked when it would be totally safe to have a colonoscopy.

6. A partner may want to watch the sex preparation. While I tend to get myself ready for partnered-sex by taking a private moment alone, I have learned that some sex partners can be fascinated by just what we do post-surgery to get it up; they may want to watch us put on those stretchy cock rings, use a vacuum pump, or even watch how we inject a prescribed erection potion.

7. Erections may take time to return with incremental gains possible. I am still waiting for more erectile success, but I did see slow progress as I approached the nine-month mark after my surgery. It makes a lot of sense that performance cannot bounce back overnight, since the nerves have been traumatized and need quite a bit of time to heal. In the first six months, erectile dysfunction pills were doing nothing for me. I decided to try needle injection medicines with the first two trial runs at the doctor's office. Neither the standard dose at the first visit nor an increased dose at the second visit made me truly hard. I had a rubbery, half-staff hose. I waited a couple of months and tried the injection at home. Bingo. I had a great erection that lasted an hour. Another month passed and I wanted to have that experience again. It was a lucky thing that I accidentally loaded the syringe with only half a dose because I was rock hard for two great hours. When I started to worry that I might stay hard too long, a shower helped me bring it down. My guess is now that the injections have proved successful a more spontaneous pill approach may be in my future, if I am lucky.

8. Maintenance medications can keep the pump going.

Some of the research is now recommending early use of the erectile drugs to get the penis oxygenated even if you don't get hard. Some of the regimens use moderate doses off and on while other regimens use low doses for a longer stretch of time. As mentioned, I had not been getting much effect from the occasional use of the larger doses, but lately I have noticed my penis at least a bit beefier using the low dose medication daily.

Getting "Out" Again

After recovery, social connections with other guys can be very healthy, too. I found it is important to find ways to network where you can explore and still feel at ease. For example:

1. Connect with other men on social levels first. I found that meeting men on a purely social level can take off the pressure of having to have sex when you are not yet up for it. Consider connecting with gay men for bike riding, theater, antiquing, and so on. And if you want to progress to something more sensual, you can tell the guy just what you are ready for. For example, you could say, "I am only up for giving you a friendly massage today."

In my own case, I advertised some simple social connections on gay Internet sites with quite a bit of success. I mentioned that I was interested in a hike, nude yoga, or even a coffee break, rather than using the typical gay vocabulary about top, bottom, and that kind of terminology.

Now, even when vacationing, I look for locals on gay sites who would be up for a naked hike along less-traveled trails. This has worked out very nicely, providing me with some gay buddies out on the trail as well as for dinners during the vacation.

2. Social nudity with other men can present some opportunities in itself. When in the locker room or out hiking nude, some men have noticed my retropubic surgery

incision and this has led them to volunteer their own prostate experiences. When a man mentions my incision, it gives me a chance to bring up what works for me and what does not due to the surgery. It is a natural way to get into the prostate topic in a relaxed style; although over time my scar is fading nicely into the camouflage of my "treasure trail," i.e., the strip of body hair spanning the region from navel to pubes.

3. A matter-of-fact attitude can make the sex go easier. I took note of a great attitude from a sporty guy I met on a gay website. The meet-up at my apartment was months before I had any inkling of my own prostate cancer. I clicked immediately with this robust guy. So while stripping off our clothes, he casually mentioned, "I had my prostate taken out a couple of years ago, so I don't shoot. I get the full orgasm but it is either totally dry or it can be a quick squirt of piss." He reached in a small gym bag and took out a piss towel and some rubber cock rings. He casually attached the stretch rings around his shaft to help him keep pumped as we got down to business. His own comfort with it put me at ease. When he left I thought to myself, "great guy!" And maybe that is how we should all approach it.

Robotic Radical Prostatectomy

Gil Tunnell

Diagnosis

It seemed like a cruel joke: prostate cancer. I couldn't believe it. At the beginning of my medical odyssey, I was in complete denial of the possibility I might have it. Like most gay men I know, I love sex. Cancer of the prostate threatened to end sexual activity completely or at least seriously compromise it. Besides, I felt youthful at age fifty-nine, exercised daily and was physically fit, felt no symptoms of any kind, and had never had any major medical problems.

The diagnostic workup began in the summer of 2008 in the usual way these things go: During a routine annual physical exam, I was informed that my PSA had shot up from 2.6 to 5.7 in the course of a year, a phenomenon called "velocity of change." My primary doctor thought I might have prostatitis (an infection of the prostate) and put me on Cipro for several weeks, but when the PSA remained at 5.7, he referred me to a urologist.

I still wasn't worried. But I did begin to read up on prostate cancer. As a psychologist, I know that people handle emotionally only as much as they are ready to. When my partner was diagnosed with prostate cancer five years previously, I read minimally about prostate cancer. With each book or essay he brought home, my anxiety mounted as I turned the pages, and I would set them aside. My partner still occasionally reminds me how I "was not there" for him initially. I was terrified for him and also selfishly for me, because we had always had a robust sex life. Even when other things weren't so good between us, sex was always an important connection.

When it came time to do my own reading as a potential prostate cancer patient, I focused, still in my denial stage, on the sections in Dr. Patrick Walsh's Guide to Surviving Prostate Cancer that emphasized how a high PSA might indicate only an enlarged prostate, which is much more treatable and is not cancer. I skittishly skimmed the next sections on prostate cancer, still not imagining that could be my diagnosis. I didn't dare read ahead about prostate cancer treatments.

In the 1980s, as a gay man, I thought AIDS would cause my death. When that fear subsided, I imagined heart disease would kill me, just as it had for everyone else who had died on both sides of my family tree. No one had ever had cancer.

During the digital rectal exam (DRE), the urologist said he felt a nodule on one side of the prostate gland, which to him suggested cancer, not an enlarged prostate. He said we needed to do a biopsy. As I told friends, the social aspects of prostate cancer began to emerge: Some friends were in even greater denial than I was. Some comments I heard:

"I would never get a biopsy at this point. There are diets that can bring down a high PSA. Take your time."

"Well, so what? If it is prostate cancer, isn't it treatable? Just get on with it."

I am a believer in Western medicine and knew I would have the biopsy; what choice did I have? Moreover, my partner, his sister (a former nurse), and my partner's nephew-in-law (a urologist) all urged me to proceed. It didn't take any special urging because my view has always been "it's better to know than not know."

The biopsy itself was uneventful. The urologist's nurse said the biopsy results wouldn't be back for ten days.

I still wasn't particularly worried. But three days later, around noon on Monday after that Friday's biopsy, I got an urgent-sounding voice message on my cell phone from the urologist to make an appointment with his secretary as soon as possible, which would be five days hence, the earliest time he would have office appointments. I was about to give a lecture to my class and wasn't able to call him back. Late Monday afternoon back in my office, I made the appointment with his secretary as he requested, but now I had begun to worry.

The urologist had told me to email him if I had questions, so I did on Monday evening. I emailed him the following: "I assume the news isn't good." An hour later he responded: "Right. The news isn't good. But we have solutions. Bring a friend or loved one when I see you on Friday."

My best female friend was furious that the doctor would send such a message via email, but it was I, after all, who had started that email exchange. I am sure the urologist wanted to see me in person rather than communicate via phone or email about the diagnosis and treatment options. My anxiety, however, was at full throttle during the five days I had to wait. I figured I did have prostate cancer; the question was what stage.

I brought my partner along to the urologist's office to hear the biopsy results. It was definitely prostate cancer, Gleason score of 3+3 (moderately aggressive), concentrated on the right side of the prostate and very near one of the two nerve bundles that control erections. As he talked, I became more and more anxious. My partner remained calm and took notes; that is part of our dynamic that has happened before. He is the calm in my storm. He freaks out later when I have my emotions back in check. But Bob had been through the prostate cancer experience five years earlier, and because he was OK now, perhaps he could be calmer about what I was struggling to absorb. On the other hand, sex had never mattered to him as much as it did to me and, at that moment, my sexuality, part of my core being, was getting a head-on assault.

The urologist continued on and recommended robotic surgery, which was his specialty, and to have the surgery sooner rather than later. No watchful waiting for me.

When I came out of my haze, I asked the urologist about the potency issue. At that point, sexual potency was my focus, not cancer control or urinary incontinence. The urologist paused and said, "I don't think I can spare the right nerve bundle, so I'd say you'll have fifty percent potency, and you'll probably need Viagra the rest of your life."

This was too much to bear, and, I suppose to break the tension, I asked, "Are you telling me I'm going to have half a dick?"

Both he and my partner laughed, but then the doctor said, "More or less."

I then became frightened as well as angry, and upon leaving the office told him that I'd be getting some second opinions. He understood. Five years before, I had liked Bob's urologist very much and immediately scheduled a consultation with him. When Bob had a radical prostatectomy in 2003, the robotic option wasn't available, and he chose to have "open" surgery by one of the top surgeons in New York City. During my consultation with that surgeon, I felt immediately at ease, particularly when he said he thought he could save both nerve bundles because of the "nerve-sparing" operation he does.

By the way, what are the odds that a gay male couple together twenty-six years would both be diagnosed with prostate cancer? We began referring to ourselves as the prostate cancer twins, saying that cancer was in our drinking water. It still felt unreal.

Decisions

I never seriously considered radiation or radioactive seeds. Friends of mine had been treated with radioactive seeds, and I had heard their horror stories. I didn't believe I would miss the ejaculate (which would be eliminated immediately if I chose surgery but not if I chose radiation), plus, at that point, I really wanted the damn cancer out of my body.

The choice for me became whether to have traditional "open" surgery or the newer robotic surgery, where the surgeon sits at a computer console twenty feet away from the patient. The robotic surgeon first places multiple (four to six) access ports across the patient's abdomen for the camera, for the surgical instruments, and for the assistant to pass sutures in and out. Once these instruments are inside the patient, the surgeon manipulates them remotely from his computer console guided by a highly magnified three-dimensional visual image of the deep pelvis where the prostate is located. The port near the naval is enlarged at the end of the operation to permit removal of the prostate gland and surrounding tissue.

My research began in earnest then. I read deeper into a Johns Hopkins white-paper report on prostate cancer and the Walsh book, and consulted in person or by phone with over fifteen gay and straight men who had been treated for prostate cancer. The myth that men don't like to express their vulnerabilities was proven absolutely untrue with the men I surveyed. I am grateful to these guys, many of whom were complete strangers who spent hours on the phone telling me about their experiences. They seemed to welcome the opportunity to talk. At that point, I began attending the monthly Malecare group for gay men with prostate cancer facilitated by Dr. Gerald Perlman. There I heard first-hand stories from men at various stages of the disease from early diagnosis and deciding treatment options (my stage then), as well as success and failure stories of the treatments they chose. Each group session was both supportive and frightening at the same time.

During this time, I learned that a straight colleague had been diagnosed with prostate cancer a year before and had just had a prostatectomy. We began talking and emailing, and he eventually became my best cancer buddy. An academic, he had already done the research, including reading actual medical journals. He sent me his reading list. My colleague, however, had chosen traditional "open" surgery and traveled from New York City to Johns Hopkins in Baltimore to have it. A year later, he was cancer free, and issues around incontinence and erectile dysfunction were resolving themselves. He seemed very satisfied with his choice of treatment.

My partner had also been pleased with the results of his open surgery, though he suffers from minor urinary incontinence, now five years later. When I had consulted with my partner's urologist, he got me nervous about incontinence, claiming that open surgery had a "somewhat" better track record here than the newer "robotic" surgery, which tended to have "somewhat" better outcomes with potency. He also reminded me that permanent daily incontinence is a fate much worse than erectile dysfunction; besides, there were treatments for impotency. He said each surgery was about equal in terms of cancer control.

I was leaning toward robotic surgery, however, but I wanted a third opinion from a different robotic surgeon. I didn't like the original robotic surgeon because he had promised me "only half a dick." Even if no one could guarantee anything, I wanted a physician who'd give me better odds, like my partner's open surgeon had already done. From my new network of cancer buddies, I kept hearing about a great robotic surgeon at another hospital, who had expert surgical skills but no bedside manner. And I got very excited when I learned my health insurance plan included him.

When I met with the third urologist for a consultation, after waiting an hour, he spent all of ten minutes with me and looked at me as though I were crazy to be even considering open surgery. He believed, however, he could spare the nerves that control potency. I also quickly told him that my partner had had open surgery and was now fully potent but had incontinence. By nature, I ask a million questions, even if I already know the answers, and I began doing this in his office. I really just wanted to get a feeling about this man who might operate on me. He stopped me, annoyed I was wasting his time, and said, "You are an intelligent man; I sense you already know your answers. Go to my website if you don't. When do you want to schedule the surgery?"

My partner was in the waiting room, and I insisted the surgeon take the time to go out and meet Bob. As he shook Bob's hand, he said, "I'm going to do a better job on Gil than your doctor did on you."

We took a cab home that evening, and I was very frustrated. I'd heard such great reports about this surgeon; I wanted to like him but the interaction left me cold. The Malecare group then became especially helpful, as several men there had had experiences with this same robotic surgeon. There was consensus: Although his bedside manner sucked, he was a fantastic surgeon.

What happened next seems minor, but it helped me make up my mind. I knew this third surgeon also liked to communicate via email, so I sent him a list of several questions, and within an hour, he had answered them all. OK, this is his preferred way to communicate. I knew then and there I'd be going with him.

To summarize, the way I saw things in late 2008, both the open and robotic surgeries attempt to spare the nerves that control potency. After removing the prostate, both procedures then re-attach the patient's urethra, which had been embedded in the prostate, directly to his bladder. Both procedures require the patient to have a catheter for one to two weeks while the re-attachment heals. Two advantages of robotic surgery are that it is minimally invasive (only four to six tiny incisions horizontally across your abdomen, rather than a huge slit vertically down your abdomen), and the operation is essentially bloodless (my partner lost far more blood than I did). Rather than the open surgeon "feeling" the prostate and the nerve bundles with his hands that inform him where to cut, the robotic surgeon remotely manipulates the mechanical surgical arms via a computer, assisted by a hugely magnified visual field so he can "see" where to cut.

This "tactile versus visual feedback" issue remains an ongoing controversy: Which source of information is more accurate in telling the surgeon where to make his cuts? Open surgery gives the surgeon tactile sensory feedback; he is actually feeling the prostate and its surrounding nerves directly with his hands. But he can't see very well because there is a lot of blood. In contrast, the robotic surgeon gets clear visual feedback from a computer screen that displays a massively magnified picture of the patient's prostate and the surrounding nerves and tissue, without all the blood. Each surgery has its proponents.

Because open surgery usually takes longer and is more physically demanding, there is the risk that the surgeon will become tired during the operation. The robotic surgeon, in contrast, remains seated at his computer console, minimizing fatigue. Also, at least in late 2008, robotic surgery required a shorter hospitalization (one day vs. three days), a shorter time with a catheter (one week vs. two weeks), and a shorter immediate recovery period (three weeks vs. several months).

Given that both robotic and open surgeries had roughly equivalent track records for cancer control, impotence, and incontinence (although robotics is relatively new, and the research can track only short-term follow-ups), I made my decision to have robotic surgery. Finally, there was the practical matter that, as a self-employed psychologist, the sooner I got back to work, the better off financially and emotionally I would be. In late November 2008, we scheduled the robotic surgery to occur December 18, so I could use Christmas vacation to recover and not miss too much work. My patients were accustomed to my taking off at least two weeks in late December. A third week would not raise eyebrows. At that point, I chose not to tell any of my patients what was happening to me medically.

In the pre-op procedures, an MRI showed that the cancer was still encapsulated within the prostate (good news), and the surgeon thought the two nerves that control potency could be spared (again good news). I was as ready as I was going to be.

I was, frankly, still more concerned what would happen sexually after surgery. I feared that the permanent loss of the prostate gland, as well as the erectile dysfunction—whether temporary or permanent—could compromise sex possibly forever. If you can't get erect, you can't penetrate anyone; if you don't have a prostate, what would be the fun of being penetrated? From the Malecare group, I learned that receptive anal intercourse after a prostatectomy remains very enjoyable because the anal sphincter is rich in pleasure-sensitive nerve endings that are not affected by the surgery.

Treatment

The day of the surgery, I met the surgeon for the first time since our brief ten-minute consultation in early November. As we were waiting for the operating room to be prepared, he seemed to tease me by asking if I had any more of my questions. I took the bait and asked him something or other. He again dismissed me. "I think you already know the answer to that; but listen, Gil, you will do fine. I am a great surgeon."

It surprised me that a patient going into major surgery actually walks into the operating room side-by-side with his surgeon. As I climbed onto the operating table, I saw the huge robotic apparatus with its octopus-like arms perched above, ready to descend onto me, as the surgeon took his place at the console twenty feet away. It was a very cold room with bright lights. The anesthesiologist and the assisting surgeons were busily strapping down my arms and inserting IV lines, and suddenly I was asleep.

The surgery began around 1:30 P.M., and I woke up two hours later in the recovery room, in horrific pain. My partner and my best female friend were at bedside and reported that the surgeon had told them that the operation had been both quick (one hour instead of the anticipated three; my partner's open surgery had taken five and a half hours) and successful in that he believed he had gotten all the cancer. He also reported to them he had "shaved" one of the two nerves crucial to potency, leaving me with one and a half nerve bundles rather than one or none.

With surgery over, recovery began in earnest. I had observed Bob's recovery from open surgery first hand; he was in a slightly weakened state for several months but generally was up and out of bed on his own right away. His particular recovery was complicated initially by painful spasms from the catheter, which his body kept rejecting.

My recovery was quite different (lots of pain in the beginning and a profoundly weakened state for two weeks, but then a fairly rapid return of energy at four weeks). Part of the difference is, of course, that we had different procedures. But even comparing patients who had the same type of surgery, everyone has a different experience.

I hadn't done my research, however, about what actual recovery from robotic surgery would involve. No one had told me that to obtain that massively enlarged 3-D visual field that informs the surgeon where to cut out the prostate and surrounding tissue, the patient's belly is filled with carbon dioxide, air that doesn't go away quickly on its own after the surgery.

In the recovery room, my belly was so enormous I thought I was pregnant with triplets. I could barely breathe. I wanted to belch and pass gas, and did so, which felt great, letting some of that trapped air escape.

I spent only one night in the hospital on the oncology unit. With a catheter in my penis and severely weakened, the nurse awakened me at midnight to do ten laps around the inpatient unit. You must be kidding, I thought. After robotic surgery, it apparently is very important to get up and start walking as soon as possible. After I maneuvered myself up with her help (it did take another person for the next few days to literally pull me up off the bed), I nodded and tried to smile at these other cancer guys doing their laps around the nursing station, all of us attached to mobile IV stands that held our medications and our catheter bags, many of us with our butts hanging out of those hospital gowns. With the trauma we had all gone though that day, no one was interested in modesty. I can laugh now but it wasn't funny then.

I was scheduled for discharge the next day at 4:00 P.M. during New York City's first major snow and ice storm of the year. The car service we had planned to use refused to be out on the streets. A friend called and urged me to get out of the hospital soon or else I'd never get home: Driving on the streets was getting hazardous. The hospital was discharging me in the middle of a major blizzard with no planned way to get me home once we got to street level! I was getting very anxious. Would the hospital re-admit a patient after discharge if there were no way for him to get home? Adding to the snowstorm problem was the dawning realization that even if we got a cab, my belly was so big I could not imagine scrunching up enough to get into the backseat. I could not bend much at all. It didn't matter once we got down on the street; all the cabs were taken. We considered taking the subway. But the closest station was several blocks away, and the sidewalks were already icy. As we were debating what to do, the transport person and Bob spied an off-duty livery limousine and hailed it. He agreed to take us for what turned out to be the ride of our lives, as the non-English speaking driver talked on his cell phone the whole way, slipping and sliding his limo on those icy streets. There was more drama yet to come, however.

Recovery

Because I had understood that recovery from robotic surgery was easier and faster than that from open surgery, I must have imagined that there would be no recovery at all. I was in no way prepared to be so physically disabled. We live in a third floor walkup apartment, and it took thirty minutes that day to climb the stairs. Once inside the apartment, I was so weak and my belly so distended (with all the air still inside) I could not bend over to take off my shoes or socks. My partner began untying my shoelaces and removing my shoes, swapped the smaller "traveling" catheter bag for the more permanent one, and went into the bathroom to empty the catheter bag.

Not only do I ask a million questions when I get anxious, I am also a control freak (no doubt the two are related). As I got into bed, I heard lots of commotion in the bathroom. I called out, "What's going on in there?" My partner slammed the door. I persisted, "What did you do? What is happening?" Bob yelled, "It's under control, leave me alone." I couldn't stand it any longer and painfully got up from bed to go see: He had somehow emptied the catheter bag from the wrong end, and urine had splattered all over the vanity, mirror, and floor. I started cursing, "Do you need a course in being a home health care aide?" He got angry. Then, simultaneously we broke out laughing, hugged each other, and I got back into bed. He may not have been the greatest home health care aide, but I realized I was suddenly totally dependent and I'd better not piss him off.

Having the catheter was no big deal. What was a big deal was my incredibly weakened physical state and needing help to do just about anything. I don't recall ever having faced such dependency; I was utterly helpless. I wasn't prepared.

Nor was I prepared when forty-eight hours after the surgery, I started having violent, uncontrollable hiccups: The carbon dioxide used to inflate the abdomen (to provide the robotic surgeon with that 3-D magnified visual field) can irritate the diaphragm. The hiccups were relentless, coming every few minutes, even during sleep. When the surgeon's nurse called several days later to check on me, she heard me having a spell of hiccups and said that is very serious and not typical. The doctor sent over a prescription for Thorazine, a major tranquilizer used to calm psychotic patients. Not only did that not work after twenty-four hours, I was now a zombie mentally as well as a mess physically. I kept trying all the home remedies for hiccups that anyone knew; nothing worked. My partner even tried to scare me by showing me a fake, inflated hospital bill.

A week after the surgery, I spent Christmas Day with a catheter in me, hiccupping. But my best female friend brought over a Christmas dinner and I had my first solid food in a week.

The hiccups continued for a solid week, 24/7. They didn't stop until my partner's ninety-two-year-old mother came to see us for a late Christmas visit. She pulled from her purse a peppermint candy and told me to suck on it. Within fifteen minutes, the hiccups stopped. I already loved my mother-in-law, but this gesture endeared her to me forever.

Earlier that day I had returned to the hospital for the surgeon to remove the catheter. He had now gotten the pathology report back from the surgery and gave me a printout, saying only, "You may need further treatment, probably radiation," without elaborating.

What? From the two-page pathology printout, I could not understand why the surgeon said I might need more treatment. Once home, I got on the Internet, and contacted my cancer buddy network to figure out what specifically in the pathology report made the surgeon say what he said; it was all medical jargon to me. I soon learned what "seminal vesicle invasion" meant: Cancer cells had escaped from the prostate itself into the seminal vesicles that line the prostate. Although the seminal vesicles are removed along with the prostate gland during surgery, the fact that cancer cells had escaped at all from the prostate automatically upgrades the patient's stage of cancer and puts him at a significantly increased risk for cancer recurrence. If cancer does recur after the prostate is removed, the only treatment options left are radiation and hormone therapy.

Doing online medical research is both helpful and scary. One medical website said patients with my kind of pathology report had a five-year survival rate. I also happened to read Dana Jennings' column in the New York Times about the hormone therapy he was then undergoing when his cancer had recurred after his prostate was removed. The online research and Jennings' essay suddenly hit me.

I closed my laptop and wept deeply and loudly. It was the first time I had been truly emotional. My cry was more like an angry wail. Damn it: I had chosen surgery to get rid of the cancer. I thought surgery was the sure-fire option for cancer control. The pathology report was totally unexpected. One lesson that I perhaps should have already learned at age fifty-nine: Nothing in life is guaranteed.

Outcomes

The surgeon's nurse called in the second week of recovery, relieved to hear that I no longer had the hiccups. I asked about the pathology report, and she confirmed that the news wasn't the greatest, but their practice tracks a "small group of men" with similar pathology reports who never have shown recurrent cancer; she hoped I would be in that group. I wouldn't know where I stood until the first PSA test six weeks later. There was nothing to do but wait it out.

Now, ten months post surgery, with checkups every three months, the PSA has remained "undetectable." Thus far, I seem to be in that "small group of men," although my PSA will be monitored for life apparently. But for now, the outcome on the cancer is very good.

What about urinary incontinence and erectile dysfunction, the two other dreaded possibilities men face after prostate cancer surgery? As far as I knew, every man who had either a robotic or open prostatectomy would need to wear a diaper pad at least for the first few months after the catheter was removed. So I was outfitted with a pad when the surgeon removed the catheter, and as we drove to our weekend home, my partner stopped twice at rest areas for me to go to the bathroom. Both times the diaper pad was dry, and I urinated normally. Bob said, "Well, I don't understand, but it will be wet later, trust me."

I have never had any urinary incontinence from the day the catheter was removed (except rarely at night while sleeping and sometimes near the end of a gym workout). To have no incontinence immediately after surgery is a minor miracle. When I emailed the surgeon to tell him the good news that I was "dry" so soon after the catheter removal, his response was, "That is great news, Gil, and a New

Year's gift from me, too. While you are thinking about it, would you go to my website and do a posting about your experience with me?" No, I thought, not so fast: The verdict is still out on cancer control and potency.

Regaining potency is a slower and very interesting process. Even if the nerve bundles are "spared" in the surgery, they are nonetheless irritated by the surgery and need time to recover. My cancer buddies had all strongly advised me to begin masturbating immediately following surgery. "You won't feel like it, but you need to do it." Even though I had zero sex drive, I dutifully started masturbating during the second week of recovery.

It was an astonishing experience to have my first orgasm without any ejaculate (though with a little urine) and with a totally soft penis. I never knew an orgasm without any erection at all was possible. It is not only possible, but in some ways it is even more powerful and enjoyable: My body shook all over, and the orgasm was more sustained than the usual kind. After several days of repeating this new experience, I noticed that my penis was getting a bit harder (my cancer buddies were right!), and I got very excited. When the surgeon's nurse called that week to check on me, I reported the good news: That morning while masturbating, I detected some hardness. The nurse literally shrieked into the phone, "Gil, stop that! You're not supposed to masturbate for several more weeks. Your surgeon has done delicate internal repair work that you could undo by 'playing with yourself.' Stop it immediately!" I felt like a Catholic schoolboy being scolded by a nun.

Convinced she was incorrect, I canvassed my cancer buddies. They all got back to me with the same message: "She's wrong. An erection is always a good thing." I emailed the surgeon with the contradictions, and his answer back was that while he was happy that I was noticing some hardness, I should lay off the masturbation for another couple of weeks.

My surgeon, who is committed to returning his robotic surgical patients back to full sexual functioning, had wanted me to take a small dose of Viagra every evening after the first few weeks, "to get the blood flowing." I wasn't consistent with that, because it made me feel flush and disturbed my sleep. For the first four months, whenever I had sex, I didn't get very erect unless I had taken Viagra or Levitra; I would have my "special" orgasms but there was no bona fide erection.

Then I discovered, somewhat by accident about four months post surgery, gay Internet porn from listening to a patient of mine. When I went to the website he had told me about, I quickly got a full-blown erection for the first time without any medication. When I mentioned this experience to my cancer buddies, they said this isn't uncommon: After surgery, intense visual stimulation may be required to get and maintain an erection, plus with visual/audio pornography there's no anxiety about "having to perform." More recently on several mornings, I have awakened with a raging erection more typical of an eighteen-year-old.

The mind/body connection in the sexual recovery has been intriguing. Before prostate surgery, the mind and body were always in synch. Now each sometimes acts independently and doesn't necessarily bring the other along. I've learned just to observe it and laugh. I can laugh because the recovery is indeed happening and the nerves are firing, however unreliably; I just need to be more patient.

Because essentially I have had good outcomes on all three fronts—cancer control, potency, and full continence—I consider myself lucky and am very thankful. Writing that sentence (and this essay), however, gets me anxious that I could jinx it all. Chance, as it is in life, is a major factor in cancer; we simply lack much control. The PSA can still go back up. Perhaps still in denial, I don't identify as a cancer patient. For now, I am a gay man who has had prostate cancer.

A footnote on physical exercise after surgery: Because I am a worrier by nature, I had fretted about the lack of exercise during recovery, not only because I enjoy exercise but also because it makes me fret less! Before the surgery, every day of my life, I had either gone to the gym, taken a long bike ride, or did yoga, all activities that prostate surgery temporarily halts. It turned out that, like many of the things people worry about, not being able to exercise for the first month was no problem at all, because I had absolutely no physical energy. However, after a month, my physical energy magically reappeared. Suddenly at four weeks post surgery, I had abundant energy, and I became impatient about being forbidden to exercise. I contacted the surgeon and he said hold off for another two weeks. Accordingly, six weeks after surgery, as with sex, I went back to exercising: gym workouts first (but no abdominal exercise because that area is still healing), then gentle yoga (to avoid stretching the tender repairs the surgeon has made), and finally bike riding (when the prostate field has better healed).

To sum up, all things considered, I have been incredibly fortunate. My body has bounced back and shown its resilience. It's amazing really, though I realize in writing this essay I have been very impatient throughout the entire process. The diagnosis, treatment, and the multiple recoveries from prostate cancer (cancer control, incontinence, and erectile dysfunction) are simply not going to happen overnight. In the immediate recovery I looked for progress daily, even though I was told to measure progress weekly. My robotic surgeon had told me that in six weeks I would be 90% back to normal. He was right. At ten months post surgery, I am 99% back.

If I had to begin the medical odyssey all over again, I would make exactly the same choices. What has been absolutely crucial in coming to terms with my cancer diagnosis and treatment has been the knowledge and support of fellow cancer buddies. This is truly a situation where unless you've been there, you can't really know. In the end, it was a good thing that my life partner had gone through it; he helped many times to "normalize" what I was experiencing. I have found that most doctors don't show real empathy, nor do my gay friends who haven't gone through the prostate cancer experience. I think it is too terrifying for them to contemplate.

But the empathy is automatically present when you talk with other men, straight or gay, who've dealt with prostate cancer. This continues to happen with my visits to my surgeon's office for the follow-up PSA blood work; men whom I don't know at all want to talk and compare experiences. The bonds are there, ready to be tapped, and it is relatively easy (given the prevalence of prostate cancer) and certainly helpful to find others in similar situations eager to start talking, either in support groups or online. The Malecare group for gay men with prostate cancer has been a place where I could pose questions I was afraid to ask the surgeon, particularly those "embarrassing" sexual questions. With the encouragement of the Malecare group, I began talking more frankly with the surgeon about sexual matters. I found I had been wrong about his bedside manner. It finally emerged when I began asking him questions I didn't already know the answers to. He was surprisingly sensitive to my concerns. I have come to like him.

At times then and now, I have been able to laugh at what was happening, and a sense of humor definitely helps but not always. Prostate cancer diagnosis, treatment, and recovery cannot help but make a man anxious. A man must confront, in my case and in most cases, suddenly, out of the blue—when he has not experienced any physical symptoms of illness and feels just fine—the very real possibilities of cancer, erectile dysfunction, and urinary incontinence. In the best-case scenario, these outcomes are temporary, but there's no guarantee that one will have that best-case scenario. If uncertainty about these possible outcomes doesn't unleash some anxiety, a man is not fully alive. I have learned to appreciate my own anxiety and understand it as an entirely normal reaction to certain life events. I have also learned the huge benefit of finding people with whom to share and bear the anxiety. Once it's shared and talked through, you can begin to deal.

Dealing with Prostate Cancer in My Fortieth Year

"James Larsen"

A Funny Bump

In 2006, near the end of my thirty-ninth year, I was lounging in bed with a fuck buddy after a very fun-filled and satisfying afternoon. Just one of those blissful moments, everything in the world was just right. And then my fuck buddy turned and said to me, very calmly and casually as he played with the hairs on my chest, "You know, I felt something up there. Like a bump or something. Maybe you should have it checked out." As nonchalant as he seemed, I knew it must be something; this fuck buddy worked in the medical profession, and he would know a suspicious bump when he felt one. I didn't panic. I didn't even worry. In fact, I put it out of my mind. That is, until the next time we fooled around and he said, this time a little more insistently, "You really need to have that checked out."

The idea of prostate cancer was not in my reality at all. It was just some vague thing that older men sometimes dealt with, not me. There was no history in my family, so I had never had any experience of any sort with prostate cancer. Well, I had heard about an uncle by marriage, not by blood, whose prostate cancer was mentioned quickly and briefly and kind of in that hushed-up tone that meant, "It's bad but he's fine so far, so let's not talk about that." Besides, my prostate felt fantastic to me.

Nonetheless, at my annual physical, I mentioned the bump, and my doctor did the usual finger exam. Now, let me get this off my chest: I don't get my thrills at the doctor's office, but through this whole ordeal I've always been a little perturbed by how quick and cursory doctors are when they perform the digital rectal exam. When I had a suspicious mole on my cheek, the doctors studied it as if some rare species of insect had been discovered and they weren't quite sure what it was. When it came to my prostate, every urologist and doctor who examined the obviously irregular quality of this so-called "bump" up in my ass spent about 0.75 seconds on it. I'm not looking to live out some doctor-patient porn fantasy; I just felt, and still feel, that if the cancer had been somewhere else in or on my body, the exam would be more comprehensive.

In any event, my primary doctor said, "Yeah, there's a bump there." My PSA came back at 0.4, so he reckoned it was probably just something unusual, a funny shape or something, but not likely to be cancer, and "nothing to worry about. But see a urologist." The urologist came to the same conclusion, that given the low PSA, my prostate was maybe just an unusual shape or density, but he needed me to come back in a couple of days for ultrasound imaging and maybe a biopsy.

I was thinking, "Wow, maybe all the sex I've had over the years has deformed my prostate. Do I have a callous?" Of course, I kept questions of that kind to myself. I mean, who would I ask? I knew the questions were silly, but still – some deep, subconscious shame came up to the surface, and I began thinking that maybe all the fun sex I'd been having was finally coming back to haunt me and this was what one got for all that pleasure.

The ultrasound couldn't determine what was going on, so the urologist took a twelve-core biopsy. The experience was unexpectedly painful; suddenly, OUCH! and WHAM! —It all started to feel very, very real and very, very scary. But I was still in denial. I remember thinking, "This is all a mistake, my prostate is just a funny shape. This is some misunderstanding, after all, my PSA is normal, right?" I went home from the biopsy and cried a little bit, which surprised me. I think part of it was the physical trauma of the biopsy procedure – it hurt a LOT, despite the Lidocaine and the doctor's assurances that I would barely feel it (I have a high pain threshold—I have several tattoos and piercings, and they never bothered me like those biopsy needles). I also think part of it was the fear, which was still under the surface, of what might be coming around the corner.

I took a long nap. When I woke up, questions were racing through my mind. What the heck is PSA? What the heck did I do wrong that got me into this situation? I calmed myself down and tried to put it out of my mind. I laughed on the phone with my best friend, as I tried to dispel the power of my freak-out by describing to him the unbelievably long biopsy needles and the nervous nurse who blanched when I jokingly reassured her that the ultrasound probe she was covering with a condom and smearing with lube wouldn't be a problem for me, but that the dozen long needles she had laid on the table were pretty intense. I waited the week for the biopsy results and tried not to think about the possibility of cancer at all; I didn't do any research, ask any questions, nothing. I was just holding my breath, holding on to the certainty that this would all turn out to be a big fuss over nothing.

I didn't hear anything from the urologist during that week, but after a few days I did get a call from my primary doctor saying he wanted me to come in to go over the results from the biopsy. Well, I knew what the results were now! If the biopsy had come back with good news, he would have said to call him, not come in. I was absolutely furious. I went to the urologist's office to get my results. He came into the exam room and asked, "How are you doing?" "I am fucking pissed off at you!" I replied, which really startled him. I was as ready as one could be for bad news, but I wasn't ready for a business-as-usual attitude.

For some reason, I was feeling really confident that I could handle cancer. I could. But I had no idea what the prostate actually did. I thought it was just something that felt great when I was getting fucked. The urologist told me that surgery was the best option for someone my age, and I asked what that would mean.

"Well," he said with resignation, "for one thing, you'll never ejaculate again."

WHAT? WHAT! That moment will stay with me forever. I felt the earth yanked right out from under my feet.

The urologist sighed and actually rolled his eyes. I guess he must get tired of men and their ignorance of their own bodies. He showed me a chart with lots of images of cancers and the anatomy of the prostate and male genitalia. It was a lot of information to take in, especially as it was given to me in a matter of about three minutes, but the gist was no more jizz. "Oh, and you might not get hard again, but no worries, you can have soft, dry orgasms." OK, I'd like to put my cards on the table here. I'm an average guy in the cock department, but I always felt that I had an ace up my sleeve—a rock-hard cock that shot a huge messy load. It was a nice surprise for my tricks, and I was proud of the big splash I would make. And now all that was going to be taken away. I didn't care at all about the fact that I had cancer, a potentially very serious one. I just wanted my boner! And my big cum-shot!

A very dear friend was waiting for me in the waiting room of the doctor's office, and as soon as she saw me, her face just fell. I told her the news as we walked out into the streets of Manhattan. We walked for a bit, and then I told her I needed to go back to work. I don't know why I did that, but I think I needed to surround myself with distraction for a while, just to keep from exploding or imploding.

I got onboard for the roller coaster ride of emotions

and information overload. OK, Gleason score of 6, a 3 + 3, two cores with cancer presence of 50%. Of course, it was localized at the position of the suspicious bump, which the doctors told me was good news. A second PSA reading came back at 4.5, but that was because of the trauma of the biopsy; it dropped again a few weeks later to less than 0.1.

Telling Others

I also had to deal with the issue of informing people who would need to know. Who to tell? What to tell? How do I discuss this information with my parent, my brothers? I was very selective about whom I told; but of those close friends and family who I did tell, most people didn't want to hear about alternative therapies or watchful waiting. Most people didn't want to hear much about it at all, given that discussing the ramifications of prostate cancer treatment options means weighing the possible outcomes on sexual performance and urinary continence. It kind of brought out everyone's hang-ups around sex, especially my straight brothers who absolutely did not want to hear about what it would mean to my gay sex-life. And they certainly didn't want to hear about continence problems.

Often, people would just try to truncate the conversation by cheerfully suggesting that a full sexual life isn't really that important. One gay friend actually said to me, "Well, you've had plenty of sex already." Oh, really, at forty, really? (It's true that I had had a lot of sex, but I had felt that the really good years were just ahead of me.)

The sudden reality of the presence of cancer in my life brought a lot of change. Relationships altered, friendships changed, and some ended when people couldn't deal with the information; at least not in the way I wanted them to. I admit my own part in those situations. One sort-of-boyfriend-regular-fuck-buddy decided about three weeks after the cancer diagnosis that he wasn't really attracted to me and never had been. I thought, "Huh. OK. Fuck you very much." Some friends were very shocked and concerned and fully present as I told them, and then disappeared completely, only to resurface months later with an "I'm a terrible friend!" email, before disappearing again. "Fuck you very much, too." This kind of yo-yo behavior in friends led me to close down and not share what was going on with some of my closest friends, which was really difficult. I just pulled away and didn't say why, because that was easier than facing the possibility of a flake-out from someone who really mattered to me.

Of course, there were also the friends and family members who completely showed up, and I am eternally grateful to them. And some fit into both camps. From the vantage point of the present, I have to say that it worked out for the best. It was hard going, because in the midst of educating myself about prostate cancer and dealing with the fear and overload and turmoil, I also had to let go of some people whom I had considered to be very dear friends.

Fortunately, I found a piece of solid ground in the midst of the turmoil. I immediately went on the Internet and found a support group for gay men with prostate cancer, Malecare, which met once a month. There I met many guys who were dealing with prostate cancer and could talk about their problems in candid terms. I'm so grateful that I live in a big city where I could find such a group. I was terrified the first time I walked into the room, and although by this point I had researched enough to expect it, it was still hard to be the only guy there who was under fifty-five. Once the guys started telling their stories, though, I knew I had come to the right place. They spoke with humor and honesty and candor, and the diversity of experiences and perspectives helped me immensely. One guy in the group was describing his problems with incontinence, laughing as he revealed the fact that he could shoot a load of piss when he had an orgasm. Wait a minute! While that might be a turn off to some guys (and I would learn over the following year that it absolutely was), I was intrigued. And, to be honest, even a little turned on.

A Turning Point

Not that it was suddenly easy, but soon thereafter came a moment when things shifted in my mind. I was walking to work through the streets of Manhattan. It was a beautiful summer morning, bright and sunny and early enough in the day that it was not too hot, and I felt very, very alive. At forty years old, I was in the best shape I'd ever been in (I'd quit smoking, was eating well, and exercising hard, getting ready for surgery but also, I think, to compensate for the coming "deficiencies" I'd have as a sex partner). I remember thinking, "Well, OK, maybe my dick won't work like it has all my life. I'm still a hot man. I'm still me. If I have to be a piss-shooting-dildo-daddy, well, that's hot too." In that moment everything changed for me. The prospect of surgery suddenly seemed less scary. The possibility of losing my hard cock and my cum seemed less terrifying and more like a challenge to be faced. A challenge I could handle. Don't get me wrong; it has not been an easy process.

The surgery was successful. I had the laparoscopic, robotic method, and the margins were good. That is, the cancer had not escaped the prostate capsule (the membrane that surrounds the prostate gland). The post-op pathology showed that the cancer was more aggressive than the biopsies had indicated, a Gleason 7, so the surgeon was really glad that I hadn't waited a year or two, which I had been considering. He was able to spare both of the nerve bundles that control erections, which had been a major concern given the size and position of the tumor (images from an MRI had shown me where the cancer was, and it was near the capsule and right at a nerve bundle).

The surgery took more out of me than I expected. I was so exhausted. I think part of it was physical, but also the emotional and spiritual toll was exacting.

Then there was the leaking. At first it really bothered me. I was leaking so much! I went through seven pads a day—on a good day. I did my Kegel exercises, and it got a little better each week. Finally, about six weeks after surgery, my doctor said I could try jerking off (he was very clear about "no orgasms" during that time, as the urethra needed to heal). At first, it didn't work at all. I couldn't get hard, my dick was leaking all the while, and I was frustrated and distracted. So I changed my approach. I designed a physical therapy for myself, a daily "cock workout." I would get my cock as hard as possible for twenty minutes at least twice a day, no matter what it took: porn, cock rings, different lubes, tying up my balls. Anything. Pretty soon, I was getting turned on despite the less-than-full erection and the dripping. Finally, I came, and came. And came! It was amazing. Not only was it a more intense and longer orgasm, I was spraying piss all over the place. And I loved it.

That was two years ago. Everything is different now. I still drip. I have to wear a pad every day now. It's much better, but it's impossible to concentrate every single minute on my Kegel exercises (which strengthen the pelvic floor muscles and provide more control over leaking). I have what is called "moderate stress incontinence." It's manageable, and I don't drip if I'm sitting still or lying down. I can sleep naked without dripping at all, which is such a huge relief. I've learned to deal with the leaking, with little tricks like "doubling up" on my pads if I'm going to be taking a long walk or a long subway ride after a couple of cocktails at a party; I now use women's pads and cut them in half, sealing the cut end with paper medical tape, so there is less bulk (and less expense). And while I'm discreet about it, I've realized that no one is paying attention when I have to show my pads to the security guards at a nightclub or the airport; they ask "What's that?" and I just tell them the truth, that I have a leaky dick because I had cancer. That shuts them up quick enough.

Those old fuck buddies? Well, let's just say they're not fuck buddies anymore. For one, maybe it was the sudden realness that the word "cancer" brought to our sexual interactions. For another guy, the thought of tasting piss made him exclaim, "Eww! Eww! Eww!" To which I replied, "Good-bye!" Another was perturbed by the mess created when I came and sprayed so much urine, thus interrupting sex to reach for towels.

I changed, too. I started craving a more genuine connection with my sex partners, so I stopped pursuing casual sex encounters. That was OK. I needed time to myself, to figure out who I was, how my dick would work, and what my sex life really meant to me. I needed time to heal physically, mentally, and spiritually, time to break old habits and start new patterns. In a way, it was like being a kid again, learning how to hold my pee, how to get hard, how to get off. When I was ready, I started dating again. Not easy; gay men my age are ready to have sex before they even know one another's names. Bringing serious and important issues like prostate cancer to the table suddenly takes the frisky online chat or casual date to a whole new level, where things are much more real and much more honest.

Not too surprisingly, in this new arena of realness and honesty, I met an incredible man who is absolutely into me—all of me. He is unafraid of the word "cancer." He respects and admires my attitude. "You own it," he says. And he loves the waterworks as well as the intensity of my orgasms. And one other thing, which the doctors neglected to tell me, but that I think all gay men with prostate cancer should know: When they remove the prostate, you DON'T lose the pleasure nerves that are stimulated when getting fucked. In fact, now I can get fucked much longer and harder than before, I guess because there's more room in there. Many men report a different, longer, more intense orgasm once the prostate is removed. I've also discovered that after I come, I can continue to get fucked (not like before, when the engorged prostate was too sensitive). It feels simply amazing. Am I looking on the bright side perhaps? Focused on the silver lining? Whatever. I can happily report that, two years after my prostate was removed, I'm having the best sex of my life!

A Sex-Positive Gay Man Compares the Challenges of Being HIV-Positive with Having Prostate Cancer and Life after it All

Lidell Jackson

As a former ballet and Broadway dancer–and a pretty good wrestler in turn–I've always prided myself on being both physically healthy and extremely in touch with my physicality. I'm also a longstanding political activist in the LGTSBT (lesbian/gay/two spirit/bisexual/transgender) community. I am also an HIV-positive, sex-positive activist who runs his own safe sex club called "Jacks of Color" for men of color and their friends. This represents more than thirty years of an adult life in which I've prided myself on being physically fit. Even as my community has weathered the horrors of an AIDS pandemic–and so many of us have seen so many of our strong, healthy gay male friends and lovers get sick and die–I've still maintained an identity of superior physical health.

During my dance years I discovered homeopathy: the science of treating diseases by administering minute doses of remedies that, in healthy people, produce symptoms of the diseases being treated, thereby causing the body's immune system to actively engage in healing itself. I particularly enjoyed the idea that my discipline and adherence to a strong physical regimen made my body an active, important partner with my homeopath in continuing to keep myself healthy.

Of course, all of this was brought into question when I sero-converted in 1991. For over eight years, I was faced with the dilemma of how my reliance upon homeopathy would keep me from progressing to a situation where I developed AIDS. I worked diligently with my homeopath to incorporate blood, colloidal, antiviral, and immune-building natural remedies into my already "hyper-disciplined" pill-taking regimen.

Alternative Healing

The summer of '99 presented me with my "Lazarus moment." After coordinating and supervising an overwhelmingly stressful camping weekend involving sixty-plus gay men, a staff, a caterer, and daily-chartered buses and vans, I suddenly developed an especially harrowing case of spinal meningitis–paralysis of my spine. This resulted in three weeks of intense hospitalization, four weeks of very confining home convalescence with hourly injections of Rocephin through a Hickman catheter in my chest, and a regimen of daily injections for a subsequent seven months to cure lingering cases of osteomyelitis and discitis in the lumbar region of my spine.

Hooked to the catheter, I felt tethered to my bed–immobile and completely useless. This was both physically and emotionally debilitating for me, not to mention dehumanizing. After more than twenty years of an exciting physical career and life, suddenly I was an invalid. Of course, I fully believed that I was going to recover, if for no other reason than I simply had the will and the resolve to recover successfully.

And I did–thanks to my personal "cocktail" of Epivir, Zerit, and Viramune, with an Amoxycillin chaser to check the re-emergence of the osteomyelitis. It was during this process that I took on the practice of questioning–and at times, countering–the opinions of my various doctors. My numerous years of homeopathy had taught me to be actively involved in, and educated about, my own sense of healing, so I wasn't about to relent now. As a matter of fact, it was here where the Internet became my friend, providing me with invaluable information on the various medications, their side effects, their combinations, and so forth. This episode served to place me on a retroviral regimen that I continue to practice to this day.

Admittedly, I regret that homeopathy wasn't more effective in fighting off the spread of the virus. However, I'm glad that at least I tried it. It was important for me to involve myself in what I felt was a natural and proactive way of trying to heal myself, rather than just relying on manufactured drugs to do the job. Somehow it seemed as if HIV had become a challenge to my system, and I had chosen to meet that challenge the best way I knew, even if I did have to finally capitulate to HIV medications to see me out of the darkness.

Another Challenge

So imagine my surprise at being diagnosed with prostate cancer in August 2001. I believe this developed as the result of a series of testosterone injections I received from my doctor between April and August of that year. Within my "sex-circuit" circle of friends, testosterone is widely used to pump up and make one feel sexier. I feel compelled to make my situation as public as possible in order to help other gay men in testosterone-driven circumstances similar to mine and to sound the alarm for them to monitor their PSA levels regularly. By the time my doctor and I checked my PSA level in August (at my own request, I might add), it was a whopping 20.5, with a Gleason of 7!

OK, on to my urologist for an ultrasound, anal probe, and biopsy. They discovered that I had prostate cancer. I suddenly found myself in the unenviable position of having to surmount yet another obstacle on the road to health. Admittedly, hearing the word "cancer" didn't seem to frighten me; after all, I'd been through the horrors concomitant with HIV, so prostate cancer seemed like a "walk in the park" by comparison.

My previous experience with various doctors around my "HIV saga" had taught me to take considerable time in educating myself about what prostate cancer is, how it develops, and how to treat it. In my humble opinion, had I been this diligent during the months in which I was receiving those lovely testosterone shots in my butt every fortnight, I might have had the wherewithal to "counsel" my doctor to monitor my PSA level more closely. Of course, I no longer receive the shots–but how I miss those "baseball biceps."

Surgery over Alternative Healing

My first inclination was to treat the cancer homeopathically with Saw Palmetto, Lycopene, and Squalene, among others. However, when my doctor informed me that I should be concerned that the cancer might spread outside the prostate, and the first place it might spread to was my back, I knew it was time for more drastic measures. After all, I had already survived that dreadful summer of 1999–and I was not about to chance having anything happen to my back like that again. I now truly believe in that old adage "whatever doesn't kill you makes you stronger."

So, as I was going into my eleventh year since sero-conversion, in February 2002, I elected to have seed implant surgery as my preferred treatment, because as a sex club owner and sex-positive and extremely sexually-active gay man, I simply couldn't afford to sacrifice either my libido or my erection; they were, and still are, both vitally important to me.

I was facing the onslaught of yet another, albeit not as frightening, disease; my original intention, to address the situation homeopathically as I had done after sero-converting a decade earlier, clearly evaporated.

The Valentine's Day seed implant surgery went especially well, with no problems at all. In fact, I was able to go in at dawn and leave by 4:00 P.M. that same day unescorted; not, however, until having to throw a veritable hissy fit after waiting for more than an hour for a changing shift of nurses, before I had to practically beg one to dislodge the Foley catheter from "my buddy." Here was yet another dehumanizing experience.

A year later, I happily found myself back to the picture of excellent health. My latest PSA was 4.5, and both libido and erection were in, shall we say, tip-top shape. Yes, there was still intermittent burning during urination. And I had become almost addicted to Flomax (which allows urine to flow more easily), especially after having missed a series of doses and having landed in the hospital again with a bladder infection that came hairs close to a renal infection. And OK, yes, my ejaculate was practically non-existent. I have, literally, "dribbles" of cum. Now, that was never really terribly important to me anyway. I always just thought of it as the sort of "icing on the cake." To me the orgasm itself was always the thing. But I used to think of it as quite "manly" to watch my eruption of loads of juice. I have learned to let go of that image of manhood.

Still, orgasms have returned intact after a slight detour. Shortly after my diagnosis, I was introduced by a dear friend suffering with the same disease, to a prostate cancer support group. I lasted barely two meetings. My being openly, outwardly, and some might say, even "frighteningly" gay was quite daunting to the predominantly heterosexual men in the room–and, who knows, I may have even caused some of the other gay men to look askance. Certainly my open admission to being a sex club owner and my avid enthusiasm for sexual freedom of expression–being both sex-positive and sexually active–

left a somewhat heavy, certainly palpable discomfort in a room where most men were more concerned about incontinence than about potency or performance.

When I discovered the gay prostate cancer support group–hallelujah! It was here where I was able to embrace, and more importantly, discuss this sexual freedom openly, as well as to compare notes on desire, potency, performance, orgasm, and ejaculate; and I stop there, because it was in this group that I discovered the concept of the "missed moment."

I knew it was happening to me–that moment while you're masturbating when you're just about to come, the physical crest of the moment, and then it subsides with nothing coming out. I actually thought it was just me until it came up in the group and several guys chimed in with their own "missed moment" experiences. I guess at that point my old resolve kicked in, and I decided that my next series of masturbatory experiences would all end in orgasm–or else! Well, I have to admit, there were some nights of close to, sometimes more than, an hour of sweat and strain. But I've jumped over that hurdle, and I'm back to my old easygoing masturbating self.

Suffice it to say this struggle to maintain my superior health and well-being had most certainly left me with a few "life lessons." First of all, I've had to become aware of the importance of my identity as an African-American gay man, a man of color, in continuing to maintain a personal sense of good health.

My several visits to both my oncologist and my urologist consistently placed me in the company of other "mature" African-American and Latino men, also in the waiting rooms, which eventually made me think, "Wow, I guess prostate cancer really does seem to adversely affect older men of color. Doesn't that mean that as older men of color we have perhaps an even more serious responsibility to pay diligent attention to our own health if we're so seemingly susceptible to this disease?"

And the answer is, yes, that is exactly what that means. As men of color, we don't have the luxury of assuming that the society in which we live is going to look out for our best interests. We really can't take anything for granted–certainly not our "assumed" civil and human rights, or that society will assist us in watching out for our own physical health. We really have to become much more proactive in keeping ourselves healthy–constantly and vigilantly watching our health and maintaining our own sense of physical security and independence.

This was somewhat of an epiphany for me–while I may have taken such reliance on physical well-being as a given when I was younger, I don't anymore. I know now more than ever that I'm not a passive partner in maintaining my own sense of well-being but an extremely active one.

Second, my experience with my various doctors has further underscored similar revelations I've had in the now more than twelve years of dealing with HIV that our doctors, unfortunately, simply don't know everything. In many instances, they know barely more than those of us who consistently take the time to search the Internet for information and process with our friends and support group partners about how to navigate the vicissitudes of having and enduring HIV and AIDS.

In their defense, it's not all the doctors' fault. They've got caseloads of patients and they are doing their best trying to keep their patients healthy. They simply don't have the time to do the research or the processing that so many of us patients do to find out how best to care for ourselves.

Nevertheless, I still think it is important whenever necessary to hold our doctors' "feet to the fire" and to challenge their decisions about our possible health solutions when we don't feel they accurately reflect our particular demographic or individual characteristics. I consistently have to remind all my doctors that I'm a gay man and that means a veritable host of different circumstances with which to contend; everything from diet to sexual practices to pill-taking regimens and discipline to, at times, specific drug and substance use choices.

Case in point: Upon leaving the clinic after my seed implant surgery, I was informed by the attending nurse about the various circumstances in which I had to be careful, since I now had radioactive iodine seeds in my prostate and perhaps my semen as well, i.e., don't impregnate women, refrain from having children sit on my lap, things like that.

I instantly countered with, "That's not at all applicable to me. What about masturbation? Am I going to have to throw away a towel immediately afterward because it has radioactive ejaculate? Just how lethal is the cum of a guy who's been seeded? Is oral and anal sex safe for or to anyone after seeding? What about all those questions?"

She replied, after closing her dropped jaw, "Well, we don't have any data on that." To which I immediately replied, somewhat smugly I admit, "Well, you should consider to whom you're speaking. I'm a gay man; I have a completely different set of circumstances here, so unless you can address those, you're not really talking to me, are you?"

Now, of course, I realize that everyone can't be as in your face as I am. But I still contend that it is about making our health care providers as educated as possible. They need to understand how we are different from heterosexuals. My feeling is that if you come across a doctor who cookie-cutters you into a category recognizable to him and thereby prescribes with absolutely no awareness of your specific, individual needs as a gay man, well, keep going until you find a doctor who will listen. After all, we really do have different sets of circumstances with which we have to contend and we as gay men deserve to be treated accordingly.

And I Thought It Was Over: An Addendum

I was extremely pleased to publish the preceding essay, originally titled "Surviving Yet Another Challenge," in the anthology A Gay Man's Guide to Prostate Cancer. It was important to me that the experiences of a mature (then fifty-four) African-American gay man surviving prostate cancer should be chronicled in the book. Moreover, I felt that my history as an HIV-positive survivor provided an interesting and important frame of reference.

But as I sit here five years later, in the emergency room of St. Luke's Hospital in upper Manhattan dealing with a bladder infection, I am faced with the reality that this prostate cancer fight is far from being over. I suppose I had been lulled into a false sense of security by what had become "seasonal" visits to my urologist and my radiation oncologist. The last two visits had yielded PSA readings of 1.7 and 1.3 respectively (recall that I was originally diagnosed in August 2001, my PSA was 20.5).

My primary care physician had switched my medication from Flomax to Uroxatral, and since early 2003 I had "weaned" myself from twice-a-day doses to once-a-day to every thirty-six hours to every forty-eight hours to what was now twice a week (Sunday morning, Wednesday afternoon). It seems in retrospect that I was being overly ambitious.

I admit that one of the consequences of surviving HIV for so many years is a tendency toward self-diagnosis. So it hasn't seemed unusual to me that I would adopt the same practice of self-diagnosis with regard to my prostate cancer. After all, I had chosen seed implant surgery over the numerous other options of treatment available—and I had seen a number of doctors before I had found one who agreed to adopt my method of treatment.

What I didn't count on was the side effects of the medications. Flomax may have served its purpose of assuring a "maximum flow" of urine through my bladder, but the attendant burning urination, occasional incontinence, and significant lack of ejaculate were all conditions through which I had to suffer for at least a couple of years after my surgery.

After taking Uroxatral for a few months, my pharmacist found a program that made the medication considerably more affordable. However, I seemed to have been under the assumption that I would eventually no longer need the Uroxatral–apparently I'm wrong. This recent emergency room visit is the second bladder infection episode I've had.

The first occurred in 2004, when I had trouble affording Flomax and spread the doses over such long periods of time that bacteria developed in my bladder. By the time I made it to St. Vincent's ER, at my primary care physician's insistence, I was so badly off that I had to be hospitalized–and was told that if I had waited just a few hours longer, I would have suffered renal failure and perhaps lost a kidney!

The bottom line is that I really thought all this time that at some point I would no longer need prostate care medication and eventually this entire "situation" would be finished. But it's becoming sadly apparent to me that I will be living with this disease for quite a while – essentially the rest of my life.

I say "sadly" because, as with HIV, I had been assuming that my prostate cancer was "chronic but manageable." However, I'm now facing the reality that it is neither. There are periods of seemingly benign inactivity interspersed with episodes of dire circumstance–so much for chronic. And although the medication is supposed to ensure maximum urine flow, I'm not certain what positive effects it has on my prostate. It's also extremely disheartening to think that this disease is manageable–only to have these episodes flare up and leave their continuing deleterious effects.

On the upside, however, there have been some benefits in dealing with prostate cancer. The most significant, of course, is that I didn't ignore the warning signs but immediately dealt with the presence of the cancer in my system. I think that years of dealing with my HIV status had laid the groundwork for that.

Moreover, I was able to make my experience public, by publishing this essay in books and by placing it on my website. This has been an invaluable benefit for the many gay men within my community who have had to deal with prostate cancer issues–and in particular, I'm grateful that so many gay men of color have thanked me for alerting them to the threat of similar circumstances in their lives. Given that prostate cancer tends to affect African-American men disproportionately more than other men, I am especially pleased that recounting my experiences here can prove to be of service.

There is also a surprising benefit from having to endure this whole ordeal, in that it has provided me the opportunity to monitor my general health much more vigilantly. Regularly scheduled doctors visits–involving everything from blood work, weight and blood pressure readings, and EKGs to the occasional CAT scan or colonoscopy–have become a necessary but not at all dreaded part of my life. As I look at my heterosexual counterparts, many of whom allow their health to decline through nothing more than benign neglect (and I include members of my biological family in this category), I feel practically blessed that I'm able to play an active role in prolonging my life.

Lastly, there is something to be said for "owning the disease." For years after being diagnosed, I saw prostate cancer as a sort of "necessary evil" that I had to endure but would eventually eradicate from my life. My new reality is that this is a disease that I have, that I've had for some time, and that I must admit is a part of my life that is here to stay. That means owning up to the disease: admitting that it exists and being realistic about dealing with it. Perhaps years of keeping HIV at bay has somehow inured me in a certain way. However, this is different. And so I'll persevere. Now all I have to do is get my PSA down to an undetectable level and then I'll be really happy.

Prostate Cancer Treatment Changed My Attitudes and Behaviors Concerning Sex

Roberto Martinez

Two weeks before I turned forty, I had a radical retropubic prostatectomy in order to combat prostate cancer. At the time it was the only choice for me, a thirty-nine-year-old Latino gay male with a baseline PSA of 7.9, a Gleason score of 6, and a strong family history of prostate cancer: one uncle with the disease and a father who had died of metastatic prostate cancer four months earlier.

I'd like to say my personal struggle was the most important thing in the world, but at that time my life and the world were both in chaos. In brief, a history of that time reads as follows: September 11, 2011 (I work a mile and a half away from Ground Zero); my father died; then I was diagnosed with the same disease that claimed my father. Terrorism and cancer were my companions.

I pondered treatment options. Seed implants were promising, but the research data covered only twelve years at most. At the age of thirty-nine, I wanted data that went back far enough to suggest that I might have at least another forty years to live. I read books and surfed the Internet for alternative treatment options. I dared to be skeptical of surgeons and the so-called "gold standard" of treatment: the surgical removal of the prostate gland. The herbal remedy I sought that would make this all go away did not exist. Even the radiation oncologist with whom I consulted said that he might opt for surgery if he were in my shoes— and he was even younger than I was. The treatment for me was clear.

In retrospect, the decision to have surgery and the resulting medical recovery were the easy parts. I had a good surgeon. He spared my nerves, so I would probably be able to feel sexual excitement and have erections. My margins were good, indicating that the cancer had not spread beyond the capsule of the prostate. Wearing a catheter was a drag, but that lasted only about a week. By the time the catheter was removed, my urinary continence was intact. I was very relieved to be feeling well and not in need of a diaper. I healed rapidly. Three days after leaving the hospital, I was walking up and down the four flights of stairs to my top-floor brownstone flat; within three weeks I was without much pain or discomfort. I felt secure in the knowledge that I had done the right thing for my long-term health. But being a sexually active gay man, the fact that I would never ejaculate again was not something even imaginable until it became all too real.

Prior to my diagnosis of prostate cancer, I had indeed been a very sexually active man. I first had sex with a man in the late 1970s while in my early teens. I first entered a gay bar in 1978 at the age of sixteen. It was a leather bar in Detroit called the Interchange. Walking into the women's room there and seeing men in various stages of what I then considered depraved and wanton sex filled me with both erotic desire and moral repulsion; it so conflicted with my Catholic school upbringing. Desire and desperation fueled my teenage sexual drive while, at the same time, I surrounded myself with school and work. I learned to veil the shame I felt about my sex life with attempts at respectability and honor. I would indulge my sexual desires later, beginning in my early thirties. In retrospect, I am glad I did.

In 1982, I fell in love with a man and realized painfully that the common materialist fantasies of having a wife and kids and a home in the suburbs would not be mine. I stayed with my lover for six years, probably longer than I should have, because we were each afraid to be alone with our desires during those first years of the AIDS epidemic. Falling in love saved me; being in Boston and not New York saved me; but mostly, being open about my feelings gave me the courage to insist on safer sex and protect myself. I was one of the lucky ones. Today, I feel I still am.

Having sex after prostate cancer is a lot like learning to enjoy safer sex. It is not the same, nor is it "the real thing." But if I wanted to enjoy life, if I wanted to have a future sex life, it was something I had to learn to appreciate. Doctors say nerve-sparing surgery preserves 60% of the nerve endings, 20% of which will grow back; yet about 20% are damaged forever, never to return. Usually, the older the patient, the less robust are the nerve endings. As my doctor said, "Is your erection the same as it was when you were eighteen? Well, sparing the nerves will not give you the erection of a teenager."

Orgasms without Ejaculation

My first post-surgical orgasm was about three weeks after surgery. I was not erect. Something the doctors and nurses repeatedly told me throughout the prep and recovery is that men can have an orgasm without an erection and without an ejaculation. Though this seemed obvious to me, as one who had experienced at least a few orgasms without ejaculation, I can honestly say that the idea of having an orgasm without an ejaculation was not once a goal of mine. After surgery, however, it was the only option.

I did not know what my life would be like without my own cum, without ejaculate. Given my sexual history, I never imagined that relearning how to have an orgasm would ever be a concern of mine. That I would have to relearn how to give myself an orgasm was more of a shock than this boy could take. After more than twenty years of sexual activity, relearning how to masturbate was a frustration, a slap in the face, a nuisance. It made me feel angry and defiant. In some ways relearning how to masturbate was the hardest thing to learn about life after prostatectomy, and relearning how to masturbate without cum was a special challenge.

A prostatectomy changes how one masturbates. It is that simple. Basic hand-to-cock stimulation does not always cut it anymore. In fact, for about four months, I barely tried to masturbate, as I was almost afraid my body would disappoint me. One morning before work, horny out of my mind, I finally lied down to beat off without the aid of Viagra or a cock ring. I slowly beat my limp dick until I finally achieved unadulterated release. It worked—that is, it relieved stress—but it fell somewhere short of expectations. Before surgery, I would think nothing of taking matters into my own hand should desire overcome me. If a quickie encounter with someone were not possible, then a quick JO would do, releasing tension and strain, and making it possible to get my mind back on work, a mortgage, or my salary. After surgery I learned that this sort of quickie was not as satisfying.

Masturbation after prostate cancer surgery demanded a total reconsideration of my erogenous zones, because stimulation of my cock and my balls alone often proved to be an exercise in futility. I know from some men that using porn increases excitement; but for me, it often exacerbated feelings of inadequacy. In my case, touch and fondling of the nipples, caressing of my body, help relax and excite me. Self-massage of arms, legs, feet, and hands go a long way in soothing my soul and nerves. Stretching of torso and limb had the effect of loosening my daily stresses and strains. Much more than before, sex and even masturbation is now about giving over of my total mind and body, not just my genitals, to fulfill a need. Previously, hand-to-cock stimulation alone was enough to light and stoke the fires, but purely genital stimulation now left me wanting. My heart and mind had to be in it or it was not going to work. Sometimes really good porn helped, but it often made me feel self-conscious. Maybe it was because I had fewer nerve endings in my nether regions. Mostly I was simply more anxious about my sexual performance period, and this alone played mind games with my sexual functioning. Whether physical or psychological, I had to come up with new techniques and mindsets in order to gain control over my new body. I had to think of new ways to smoke out negativity and focus concentration on the desire to make sexual activity worthwhile again.

Nor can sex with a partner be tied to a kind of checklist of stimulators that once worked so easily. Time, preparation, and foreplay are paramount. Quality body-time is key. This is as true in my own masturbation as in sexual relations with a partner. The days of rushing to jerk off to release frustrations are mostly over. Like bad sex, a lousy masturbatory experience is usually not worth the time it takes to shuck your shorts. After prostate cancer, bad masturbation defeated me on multiple levels, reminding me that the plumbing had changed, that I could no longer shoot—often discouraging me from taking matters into my own hands.

There is no cum anymore. The first few months of learning about and getting used to my new body, it was repeatedly shocking to masturbate myself to a pleasant orgasm, for I had no visual cue to affirm my orgasm. Having an orgasm was generally not a visual experience after surgery. Yes, I had the tightening of muscles and balls. Yes, I can have a moment of great release. But now the amount of work necessary for this sexual experience is greatly increased. Of course I can still come. I just don't shoot anymore and this is new and permanent.

Sometimes when my orgasm was not that strong, I wondered if I had really come at all. Had I faked it? Or had I just gotten myself really, really aroused, so much so that even my little pre-orgasm was almost enough for me? I never imagined before that it could be possible for a man to even fake an orgasm, but given that no ejaculate is present, it is technically possible to fake one's own orgasm. On at least a couple of occasions, I had to be content with just getting really close yet never finishing it off. From my own standpoint, it's not worth the trouble. What is the point of faking your own masturbatory orgasm? Perhaps one's security in this comes with age, saying it's OK to just be held and intimate and not come. Perhaps it is OK to just be aroused and not really shoot. Sometimes it just feels like a premature ejaculation under your own skin. It's as if one came slightly but it was not really satisfying. Premature ejaculation without cum is particularly confounding. I wondered, "Did I come too soon? Did I come at all?"

Anonymous sexual encounters can be great, but they are often fraught with different stresses. On more than a few of occasions, I've had a wonderful sexual encounter with a relative stranger only to have my sex partner interject, "Wow, you did everything but come." Ninety percent of the time it is not worth discussing post-coitally; but at other times, I find that sexual intimacy begets a desire for further closeness. On occasion, I've volunteered sheepishly afterward that I was sorry I didn't come. I allowed that I had cancer a few years back, only to have the guy retort, "Huh, I didn't even notice." Sometimes I feel that men can be such pigs.

Occasionally, I've tried to explain online, before I meet someone, that I had cancer and though I can have an orgasm, I can't ejaculate. That approach usually works only for people I've had some online rapport with over time. However, usually in a moment of compelling passion, I find there is seemingly no point in going there. The aim for me is to reach the point of no return in the bedroom, not to reach that point before I connect.

Changing Views and Experiences of Sex

A prostatectomy changed how I had sex. I notice now that I have about two or three different kinds of orgasms. I can still have a mind-blowing orgasm, and that is absolutely the best news of all. The tensing of all bodily muscles, the mental focus needed to make sex successful; these are all things that happen more frequently with my current domestic partner and no one is happier about that than I. Even a mediocre orgasm can be better than previously because, before the surgery, the aim would have been merely to bust a nut. Now the aim is not only to bust a nut, but also to convince myself that it is worth the half hour of planning needed for Viagra to kick in, or to wear a cock ring, and/or to suppress any fear of performance anxiety I might have. As for a weak orgasm, it is almost not even worth going there at all. I notice that I tend to "save" it a lot more than I used to, but I don't know how much of this is a factor of getting to be more middle-aged and how much of it is the new plumbing.

A prostatectomy changed how I think of sex with my partner. Talking with a steady partner and taking time and planning sex makes a world of difference. If anything, I've noticed that sex with my partner is more valuable for me. Maybe it is because having a steady partner takes some of the guesswork out of negotiating my body. Maybe it's because my partner knows over the long term how best to please and be pleased. Maybe it's because once you have a partner who helps you through cancer you realize what their true mettle is, and that this is more valuable than any orgasm alone.

A prostatectomy changed how I think of women, mostly in terms of what works for me sexually; the caressing, the touch, the time, and the trust sound vaguely reminiscent to how women often talk about "making love." It is a complete and total body experience, maybe involving

243

evolutionary desires to be protected and procreate. Perhaps that lack of an external indicator of sexual release (cum/ejaculate) makes the concentration of desire a much more worthy goal. Men can always look to a visual frame of reference for physiological completion. For me, after a prostatectomy, it is no longer a simple visual frame of reference that produces knowledge of my own pleasure. It is not something external that validates your claim to an orgasm. Sex for a man after prostate surgery, at least for me, has validity only when it is internally valid. External validation is limited to an erection alone.

Prostate Cancer and Aging

Sex after prostate cancer is implicitly connected with getting older, and at age thirty-nine, I definitely had to confront the shock of aging at an earlier age than most of my peers. A friend with prostate cancer who is even younger than I am said that he felt he was kicked into instant middle age with his diagnosis—and he is right. I developed some strong connections with men in their sixth and seventh decades of life, and now I had more in common with other men who died in their seventies. I no longer easily discount the feelings of older men. A greater appreciation for older men went hand in hand with my experience with prostate cancer.

My midlife crisis occurred when, at the age of thirty-nine, I realized that I had more in common with the average sixty-year-old man than I did with my own peers. I immediately felt this incredible kinship with older men, as they were the only ones who seemed to know what I was talking about. Men's understanding about prostate cancer seemed directly proportional to their ages; the older they were, the greater the level of the understanding. Some younger men had exposure to people in their own families with the disease. However, on the whole, this was not something I expected most men in their thirties to even care about, much less know. I think a few men who were in their twenties and to whom I spoke honestly about my cancer seemed almost afraid of me as though I were an old man! Sure I was angry for a while about feeling old, but in the grand scheme of things prostate cancer is a good cancer to have. A great deal is known about how to reduce complications and to extend one's life. And it is a relatively slow-moving cancer. After seeing children with cancer in my trips to my oncologist, children who had never lived a life, I knew how relatively lucky I was.

Support

In the days after my prostatectomy, I went to a gay male prostate cancer support group to help sort out my thoughts, and most days discussions centered on the disease and its cure. But after a relatively short period of time, I was most interested in focusing on the emotional dimensions of my sexual future; perhaps it was because, like many in this community, I had a close relative with the disease. That my sexuality was so important to me made me painfully aware of how my father's experience with prostate cancer must have been. In the months after my surgery, I met many men who had the same consequences with their prostate surgery as my father had. His operation in the late '80s predated today's nerve-sparing techniques, and he suffered from total impotence for the last fifteen years of his life. In the group, men would speak of their own struggles with impotence; and in their anger and frustration I heard my own father speaking to me from a world beyond.

How I wish I could have talked to him from my current perspective. Oh, the questions I would ask, or wouldn't ask. My father lacked much formal education and was fatalistic. When he was given his diagnosis of cancer,

245

he said it was as if someone had stabbed him in the back. Still, in his silence and pain, I would want to know: Did you know you would be impotent before you had surgery? How long did it take for you to come to terms with it? Did you have other friends who went through this with you, or did you keep it to yourself? Did your faith in God help? How did my mother help? How did your former mistress help? Is that why you supported me in front of Mom in my desire to go out at night? Did you want me to know that someone could enjoy the fruits of manhood? Still, these questions went unasked, unimagined even. My father was a man obsessed with his own mortality. We once traveled throughout Mexico in 1974 because of a dream my father had that he would die that year. My father had been planning for his death for at least twenty-five years before it happened. When it finally did happen, my siblings all gathered and said, "Well, this is finally it." Little did I know I would think of him every single day for more than a year after my own treatment for prostate cancer. My closeness to him in death made it difficult to be surrounded by men in the same circumstance.

After a couple of months, I could not go to certain meetings because of their emphasis on complex major health problems and my seemingly self-centered focus on my minor surmountable ones. I lived in a new age: the age of Viagra, an age that eerily coincided with the post-9/11 world. I have no ejaculate, but I do have erections, medically-induced or enhanced if necessary. So, all is not lost. I cannot go back in time, and I cannot spend time contemplating the past.

Ten Years Later

Anniversaries are powerful events, and the tenth anniversary of 9/11 was a fitting time to revisit the preceding essay. In the last year alone, Osama Bin Laden was killed, and the National September 11 Museum & Memorial at the site of the World Trade Center was finally finished. Some things do take a decade. In the intervening ten years, I am over most of the shock and awe regarding my illness, and the preceding essay, which appeared in A Gay Man's Guide to Prostate Cancer, was as much an effort to make sense of a world changed forever.

I worked a mile and a half away from the World Trade Center where the smell of burning steel and plastic lasted well through Thanksgiving. The 9/11 anniversary brought other vivid memories, like travelling on an airplane a mere week after the barbarism to visit my father in Detroit, who was dying of prostate cancer. It would be last time I saw him, for he died three weeks later. I had wanted to cancel the trip, but the airline would not let me reschedule unless I gave them another date. During the week of his wake, the anthrax scare was in full-bloom in the subways and on the streets of New York—I saw the reporting on CNN from the funeral parlor. Rarely have I been so relieved to be in Detroit.

As I write this, the PSA test is under attack by the United States Preventative Services Task Force, which argued that over-treatment and over-diagnosis is causing needless biopsies and surgeries that cause incontinence and impotence. In explaining my illness and treatment, I've encountered people who had stories to tell about themselves or their fathers having high PSA numbers and therefore having repeated biopsies with the result being no cancer was found. In response, I tell them the PSA saved my life. An acquaintance, an African-American law professor with no family history of prostate cancer, had a PSA of over 50 when he was first tested at age fifty, a PSA already too high for surgery or seeds. He died in his early fifties. A co-worker I've become acquainted with had such a high PSA a year after surgery (a Gleason 7) that he was told he had five to seven years left to live. He is also in his early fifties. I need only be reminded of their plight to realize their predicament could most certainly have been mine. I hope that they continue using this test until a better test is found, at least for men in high-risk groups.

I am planning on having a big party for my fiftieth birthday this spring, as it also celebrates exactly ten years since I was diagnosed and treated for prostate cancer. I think I've finally begun to experience the slowing down of my sex drive as I get older, but that has occurred only in the last few years.

Of late, I've shared this essay with a variety of men and women, but particularly with gay men dealing with a variety of prostate concerns, and not just cancer. From the Malecare support group, I learned how Flomax and similar medications can cause retrograde ejaculation (the semen goes into the body rather than out of it) and how many urologists presume heterosexual activities and downplay any discussion of these effects. A friend remarked that no one writes or talks about how sex changes for middle-aged men, and particularly how sex changes for middle-aged gay men. To do so seems to invite visual comparisons to being just a dirty old man, and in our community we avoid those comparisons.

My greatest satisfaction has been receiving the responses of a few readers who've contacted me out of the blue to tell me how helpful my essay was to them. Getting fan mail at work was something I never expected. Equally gratifying has been my sharing this with a few sex educators, one of whom has assigned this essay to his online class. I was happy when young readers thought that developing intimacy and using erogenous zones that men don't even think about was important. How prostate cancer can change one's sex life from one of genital stimulation and ejaculation as the only markers of sexual fulfillment to one where the full body must be engaged.

But my essay was not received by the class without

criticism. One female student felt I vastly simplified female orgasms, pointing out that many women have difficulty reaching orgasm or knowing when the full orgasm has occurred. She noted that, "The female orgasm is much more complicated and difficult to attain than the male orgasm, especially with a partner." Another student disliked my alluding to 9/11. All I can say is that in those days and that year it all melded together for me. Cancer does not have good timing.

Learning how to continue to grow sexually will definitely be a challenge for the next few decades, and frankly, I'm looking forward to it. I would be the luckiest man in the world were I to get a chance to reflect again in another ten, twenty, or thirty years.

Treating Erectile Dysfunction after Prostate Cancer Surgery
A Gay Man's Experience of Getting a Penile Implant

Joe Davenport

A Kick in My Gut

The first step in my journey with prostate cancer began with a visit to my primary care physician in January 2007. I had a stabbing pain in my lower back, which my doctor suspected was a kidney stone and referred me to a urologist. The urologist confirmed that I had a kidney stone, but as part of the exam, he did a digital rectal exam. He assured me that my prostate was "nice and smooth." However, blood tests revealed an elevated PSA of 4.2. He had me back in for a biopsy, and this had me concerned.

I was a relatively healthy, robust man of sixty-three, despite having been treated for diabetes, high blood pressure, high cholesterol, and HIV. Although I was on top of these medical conditions, I guess I was naive about prostate cancer. I wasn't 100% sure what the prostate gland actually did and the doctors didn't do a very good job of educating me. I wasn't prepared for how unpleasant the biopsy was, nor for the bloody ejaculate following it that lasted several weeks.

I got a call from the urologist a week later on a Friday afternoon. My office was hectic, and I did not return the call until the following Tuesday. When the doctor did reach me on Wednesday, he told me bluntly over the phone that the biopsy revealed I had prostate cancer, with a Gleason score of 7 (3+4), which meant the cancer was moderately aggressive. It was like a kick in my gut.

When I met with the urologist the next week, he emphasized the "good news" that there were "lots of treatment options," and led me to expect that I would be treated and make a full recovery. He presented all the options to me: radiation alone, radiation combined with radioactive seeds, surgery (which he questioned as a good option for me because of my HIV status), and finally watchful waiting. I expected the doctor to lead me through these choices and help me reach a decision. Nope! I was on my own apparently. Over the next two weeks, I saw three oncologists, hoping to get some direction. I discovered that while there are many options for treating prostate cancer, there is not much help in making that crucial decision. I finally found one doctor who would voice an opinion, and I chose to have a radical prostatectomy, which he recommended.

Once the treatment decision was made, I began to feel a whole lot calmer. I believed I would not die from this thing. My attitude was it's serious but I'll be treated, I'll heal, and then get on with my life. I told myself, "This is 'only' prostate cancer." I had read that prostate cancer was considered the "good" cancer because the cure rates were very high. Back then I arrogantly referred to my cancer with a small "c" because it shouldn't merit the same severity as the "bad" cancers, such as pancreatic, colon, lung, and so forth. I have come to learn there is no such thing as a good cancer or a cancer that doesn't merit a capital "C." They all suck; some just suck more than others.

Going into this journey, I felt strong and hopeful and fortunate that I did not have to go through this alone. After all, I was surrounded by good friends and family, and especially by Don, my loving partner of eighteen years. And the doctors had assured me I would be treated and cured.

My first consultation with the surgeon was at the same

famous cancer treatment hospital where my little brother had died at age twelve many years ago. Going through those doors made me pretty emotional, as I pictured my poor mom sitting there registering my brother, signing all the papers obligating her for bills she could never pay. But she did it, and with Don at my side so did I. We decided that I would have a robotic laparoscopic prostatectomy to remove the prostate gland completely and hopefully all the cancer. We set the date for June 26, partly because Don, a third grade teacher, would be off for the summer and thus be better able to look after me.

Radical Laparoscopic Prostatectomy

I went to the hospital that day at 5:45 A.M., and was in the operating room by 7:00. I understand the surgery started at 8:30, but I was snoozing by then and woke up in the recovery room in early afternoon. I was told that the surgeon found exactly what he expected and there were no surprises. The doctors felt that they were able to spare the nerves that control sexual functioning, and if everything healed as it should, I'd be as good as new. Well, maybe not as good as new, but as good as a sixty-three-year-old man should expect to be. Everything about the hospital was top notch, and when I returned home I was up and around in a few days. In early July, I returned to the hospital for what I call my own Independence Day: to remove the catheter. The hospital had gotten the pathology report back by then, and I learned that the cancer was more widespread than the biopsy had revealed (all four lobes of the gland instead of two, suggested from the biopsy, had been involved) and that cancer cells had penetrated the capsule to the layer of tissue that surrounds the gland (the surgical margin). But they had removed that tissue, too, and found that there was no cancer in the lymph nodes. The doctors were quite certain they had gotten all the cancer. It was a good day.

They fitted me with some disposable underwear that they said might come in handy.

Cancer-Free, But Incontinent and Impotent

Little did I know how "handy" the underwear would be and how long I would be wearing them. Somehow I thought that when the catheter came out, my plumbing would go back to normal with only an occasional mishap. There is something very emasculating for me about wearing a diaper. To add insult to injury, the directions for the generic pads say to insert them "into a pair of close fitting panties," another shot to my masculinity and dignity. I am a bit of a control freak, and not having control of this most basic bodily function was annoying and frustrating. In the beginning, I went through fifteen pads a day, plus an extra diaper at night, and slept on top of a towel and waterproof pads. I had some bad days in those first two months. It taught me not to take life's small conveniences for granted again. By the end of that first summer, I felt as though I had aged ten years in three months. I had never felt old before this, but I sure did then.

By October, four months post-surgery, I was still dealing with bladder control and was told the lack of control might continue for as long as eighteen months. I suggested that my friends should invest in Depends stock. I continued to wear one to three pads during the day, and doubled up at night, but the occasional accidents had stopped. Of course, I was anxious to get to the point where I didn't have to wear any pads at all. Would I ever get there? The literature warned me about incontinence after surgery, but I thought it applied to older or less vigorous men, certainly not me. Being patient is not one of my stronger qualities. I wasn't in any pain at all, but it was very distressing to lose control of this basic bodily function.

However, soon I was facing something even worse

because it might not ever improve, and that was my impotence, although the medical term of erectile dysfunction (ED) sounds so much nicer. The oral medications such as Viagra weren't helping, so the doctors wanted me to start a series of penile injections: OUCH! The doctors seemed confident they could get my sexual potency back to normal within eighteen to twenty-four months.

The penile injection hurts about the same as any injection, which is to say not much, but the conditions under which they administer it were very unpleasant. I met with a male nurse practitioner, who I think was gay. I was placed in a small, sterile hospital room and instructed to change into a hospital gown. The male nurse came back with the syringe and checked me out. Things were pretty normal; at least he didn't run from the room screaming or laughing. He gave me the injection and left me alone for about ten minutes and told me to "try to arouse myself." When he came back, I think he was pretty disappointed in my reaction, which was nil. I was lying down, which I learned affects blood flow, so he told me to sit up and try again. He came back after another ten minutes and asked me to rate myself on a scale of one to ten, with six being firm enough for vaginal penetration, and eight firm enough for anal penetration. I didn't ask him what I'd do if I had a ten. I could see some slight improvement, but certainly no gold star. At one time I thought my worst nightmare would be to have someone change my diapers, but I never envisioned someone rating the quality of my erections. Maybe it wouldn't have been so bad if I had scored a ten, but I didn't even come close to a six. I can't tell you how humiliating it was to have another man test your virility and to fail the test.

I kept up the injections with very mixed results. I was beginning to question my choice of having prostate surgery. In late fall, I started going to Malecare, a support group for gay men with prostate cancer. I wish I had gone to this group earlier; it helps hearing experiences from others in similar situations.

Even though I was continuing with the injections, I was not improving like the doctors expected. Doing the injections was very difficult for me, and then not getting good results really began to get to me. The hospital referred me to a psychotherapist, who turned out to be very helpful, just to get all this off my chest. He also gave me helpful medical information.

At this point when I went to the support group, there was a constant refrain heard about the table: be patient. I heard that from my therapist, from my regular doctor, and from my partner. So I tried. This process was akin to watching grass grow except grass grows faster. Finally, by early January 2008, with the help of a new medication, my plumbing had improved greatly: I told my friends they should not let me sit on their fine upholstered furniture, but I could be trusted on a hardback wooden chair.

Permanently Impotent?

In February 2008, I had a personal meltdown. When I met with my ED specialist, he gave me news that, for me, was absolutely devastating: That I wasn't making any progress toward getting back an erection. I had developed a venous leak, and there wasn't any hope that it would improve—I was impotent. A venous leak is when the veins that carry the blood out of the penis, which are supposed to close tightly during an erection, don't close well enough, so the blood flows out and you lose your erection. To say this was disappointing would be putting it mildly. While I was appreciative that I appeared to be cancer free, it did not come without a hefty tab. Admittedly, this is a quality-of-life issue, not a life or death one, but the possibility of being permanently impotent struck me at my very core. I was somewhat ashamed at my own reaction to this news which caused me to crawl into a fetal position and cry like a baby. I was an emotional mess for the first couple of weeks, and the only one I could discuss the situation with was my partner, who held me when I cried, and cried with me when I couldn't be consoled. He refused to accept the doctor's prognosis and had more confidence in my ability to recover than I did.

The Malecare support group suggested I get another opinion from someone who might offer more hope. I went to another hospital and met the first urologist I have actually liked. Maybe it was what he was telling me: He offered much more hope and said I would continue to recover over the next twelve to eighteen months. At that time, I actually believed that the truth lay somewhere between these two opinions; I would not be permanently impotent, but it's going to take longer than eighteen months. Unfortunately, both the new doctor and I were wrong—I did not recover.

I was also distressed that I still didn't have complete bladder control, but I did start going "Commando," or trying not wearing a pad at all to see what would happen. I can't tell you what a wonderfully freeing experience it was not to wear a pad. I still had some leakage without a pad on these "experiments," but they gave me hope that one day I could be completely free of the pads.

In August, I had my annual meeting with my laparoscopic surgeon. It was the first time I'd seen him since I had become aware of my long-term prognosis on ED. He seemed quite surprised that I was not absolutely thrilled with my recovery. He was quick to remind me that my PSA was still undetectable. I was very appreciative of that, but I wished he had been more upfront with me before the surgery about my prospects for a complete recovery beyond being cancer free. He had plenty of reasons now for why this did not go as expected—none of which had been discussed before surgery. I was angry.

On January 9, 2009, I wrote a friend: "It is apparent to me that I am not getting any better and probably won't heal much more. It seems my recovery is just about complete, and I have reached a plateau at a much lower level than anyone expected, especially me. I thought that after surgery I would bounce back and be my normal old self again. Nope. It appears that I am cancer free and for that I am very, very grateful, but there are no free lunches. Everything has its price. My incontinence is much improved with the new medication. Except for coughing or sneezing, I seem to have my plumbing under control again, finally. But I still can't get an erection. Don reminded me of the AA acceptance prayer from time to time until it began to make sense. It was a very tough pill to swallow, but what choice do any of us have? Shit happens. Now, thanks to a whole lot of counseling, some happy pills, and the support of the best damn boyfriend in the world, it looks like I am adjusting to "my situation."

Well, yes and no. I was trying to adjust but wasn't there yet. I had done everything I was told to do and more, confident that, if I were a good patient, things would turn out well. I went back to work and tried to go back to my regular life. But it seemed that I would never be my same "old" self again. These "little" problems had ballooned into major problems for me physically and emotionally. The ED issue became more complicated than the incontinence issue. I have spent more time crying over this single issue than I have in dealing with all the losses in my life combined, which then just adds more guilt and shame to the mix. Fortunately, I have a terrific psychologist who listens to me whine and cry almost weekly, constantly assuring me that the depression would pass and that I still had options. Those little blue pills did not get me back in the game, nor did the penile injections, which I did faithfully three times a week and hoped for the best. All I can say is that the best didn't happen.

The Decision to Have Penile Implant Surgery

In April, my ED specialist started talking more seriously about my having surgery to install a penile implant. In this surgery, plastic tubes are inserted down the length of the penis, along with a small sack of fluid in the pubic area, and finally a little pump with a valve that goes into the scrotum, like a "third ball," which when manipulated inflates and deflates the penis with the fluid. The ED specialist had brought up this option before, but I kept rejecting it because for the longest time the doctors thought I'd get better without it. But my situation had changed. Without the implant surgery, I would never get back even close to my "old" self again. It is my nature to do all I can to fix a problem and then move on.

So, on April 9, 2009, with Don beside me again, I was back at the hospital for what I hoped was my final surgery. It was a very short procedure, completed in less than an hour, and my surgeon is one of the best. I was out of the hospital in a few hours. I was cautioned that I would have considerable pain, and I came home loaded up with Vicodin. Well, it turns out I am blessed with my dear mom's tolerance for pain because I had virtually none. I popped a couple of pills the first day in the hope of staving off the pain, which thankfully never came. Recovery was uncomfortable and inconvenient, but almost pain free.

When I returned to see the implant surgeon two weeks later, he was astonished by my recovery. He said in thirteen years of doing these procedures I was the first to report a pain-free experience not requiring painkillers. He asked me if I was just a tough guy. I have to admit that felt good to hear. Believe me, I hadn't felt very tough in quite a while. I hardly even felt like much of a guy at times.

Recovery from the penile implant surgery took four to six weeks. After that, the doctors encouraged me to start using my "new equipment." That first weekend when I tried it on my own, I became more and more uncomfortable as the long holiday weekend progressed and couldn't wait to see the surgeon on Tuesday to ask for the implant to be removed. Apparently I was successful at inflating the device, but didn't do a very good job at completely deflating it, leaving me with an uncomfortable appendage for most of the weekend. But they retrained me, and I can now inflate and deflate the penis properly.

The new equipment works fine and is better than nothing, and it has helped me a lot mentally. But physically it's been a bit disappointing because nothing works as well as the original equipment. I always feared I might have to get used to false teeth someday or maybe a hearing aid, but never this. Yet, I know people with false teeth and hearing aids who seem to have adjusted nicely so…?

At the end of the summer, we went on a three-week vacation and I never thought about this stuff, not once! Within a couple of days of returning, however, I was back seeing doctors and starting to fall back into the same funk. I think it's time for all this activity to recede into the back of my mind and replace it with more productive stuff. That's my goal now.

I am weaning myself from the doctors. I had a visit with my incontinence doctor and I don't have to see him again for six months. That situation isn't perfect, but it's much better. I see the implant doctor next month and hopefully don't have to see him for a while. That just leaves me with the psychologist who has guided me through much of this. Little by little I am freeing myself from the doctors, and the further away from them I get, the happier I seem to be. They have all done what they can, and for that I am very grateful. Now it's time to move on and not have the cancer experience be the center of my life. I will continue with my support group once a month and hope for the best.

Like the rest of this prostate cancer journey, each individual is different, will make different treatment choices, and will have different outcomes and side effects. I now understand the reluctance of doctors and others to give advice on the choice of treatment. One size certainly does not fit all.

My View on the Implant Six Months Post-Surgery

Someone recently asked if I would have the implant surgery if I had to do it all over again. This is a difficult question with which I have wrestled continuously since the surgery. The answer is complicated and cannot be answered with a simple yes or no. My answer changes almost daily.

Once it was determined that I was impotent and would probably remain so for the rest of my life, I spiraled into a deep depression, going to bed crying and waking up many mornings with tears in my eyes. I had all this sadness and grief, even with the support of a great partner, my regular psychotherapy sessions, and taking anti-depressants. I have had some very deep personal losses in my life, but nothing compared to my reaction to being left impotent. I was embarrassed, angry, disappointed, sad, but most of all, I felt ashamed—ashamed at my reaction to what some would consider a relatively minor quality-of-life issue, ashamed that being cancer-free wasn't enough. I see people every day carrying burdens so much greater than mine, and I am ashamed of my sniveling, girly-boy feelings about all of this.

As my partner has pointed out, for me it really wasn't a choice. I had tried everything to get back to my "old" self and to be sexually functional, but nothing had worked. I wanted to be my "old" self again and an implant seemed to be my only hope. I hoped the implant would make me feel better physically and emotionally. I was a sad, emotional mess, not suicidal but there was no joy in my life.

It's now six months post-implant surgery, and I remain ambivalent. Emotionally, I feel so much better, an improvement that began the very day I went home from the implant surgery. I don't know what the connection between my psyche and my penis is, but I do know that there must be a very strong bond there. I felt stronger, better, more confident, and a bit manlier. This reaction was immediate and has never changed. Emotionally, I am much, much better.

However, physically my reaction is dramatically different from what I had expected. My first disappointment was the realization that my penis would never be totally flaccid, and that I would be blessed or cursed with a partial erection 24/7. The surgeon had told me that with the implant, even when deflated, my penis would still be about two or three in hardness on the ten-point erection scale. I had envisioned that a two or three would leave me in an unnoticeable, although somewhat engorged, flaccid state. While I'd never object to having a more robust looking penis, I think I actually have what I consider to be a constant four or five. This state is not totally uncomfortable, but it makes it hard to forget you have an implant and requires you to approach subway turnstiles and young children with some caution.

Does it work and does it feel natural? It works wonderfully. A firm erection can be achieved each time and will last as long as you like. What's missing is the sensual excitement of achieving an erection as a build-up process. With the implant, an erection is either there or not there. The erection happens quickly as soon as you squeeze the third ball in your scrotum. I miss the sensuality of the build up much more than I ever thought I would.

Perhaps over time activating my new equipment can be incorporated into foreplay and be part of the lovemaking. But at the moment switching the implant to "on" seems an uncomfortable intrusion and a reminder that I am different than I used to be.

All this said, my answer right now is, "Yes, I'd choose

to have the implant if I had to make the decision again." Especially after the delightful evening my partner and I shared last night. Maybe I am now coming to terms and accepting my situation, hopefully letting it recede to the back of my mind. Only time will tell.

A Good Outcome to My Experience of Penile Implant Surgery

Frank John

The Beginning

My story has a good ending, but it didn't start out well and has had a rocky course. I was fifty-two when I was diagnosed with prostate cancer. The first indication something was wrong occurred nine months before the official diagnosis. During a routine blood examination before some surgery to repair a torn rotator cuff, my PSA came back 9. After the shoulder surgery, my doctor did a prostate biopsy, which detected no cancer. He then put me on various antibiotics to try to bring the PSA down.

But after nine months of watchful waiting, the PSA was not coming down, and the doctor refused to do another biopsy. I had had a difficult, two-week recovery from the first biopsy, and the urologist didn't want to put me through another one. He advised me to continue the watchful waiting and to take antibiotics. I was losing patience and I didn't like the idea of taking antibiotics indefinitely. Having had the prior nine months to speak to various doctors and do research on prostate cancer, I knew that when caught early, prostate cancer was very treatable. However, I also had learned that almost all of the various treatments available can cause some degree of sexual dysfunction.

So I sought a second opinion. My PSA had gone up to 11. The new urologist did the second biopsy, which confirmed stage II prostate cancer, i.e., cancer was confined to the prostate gland, detectable via a PSA blood test and/or digital rectal exam, and involved in a single nodule in one lobe of the prostate.

Back then, I thought to myself, there's got to be a reason why this is happening. I'm not religious, but I am spiritual. The cancer diagnosis became a wake-up call to change my lifestyle, but I was heartbroken at the thought that my sexual function might be compromised. As a sexually active gay man, my sex life was very important to me and a very big part of my life. I was proud of my body, my penis, and my erections. This was a large part of how I defined myself.

The second urologist recommended robotic surgery. He was a good salesman. I liked the ideas of a less-invasive surgery and a faster recovery time. Knowing I'd have side effects from either surgery or radiation, why not bite the bullet, I thought, and opt for the surgery and get rid of the cancer? I've lived with cancer in my family for a long time. My sister was diagnosed with Hodgkin's disease and told she had five years to live. That was thirty-eight years ago and she is still alive, but the idea of cancer hangs over my family.

Soon after my diagnosis, I went to the Malecare group in New York City, a support group for gay men with prostate cancer. I remember that night so well. I was crying in the group. My biggest problem with treating prostate cancer was the possible side effect of losing my sexual potency. Some of the men in the group that night seemed resigned to losing theirs. I also heard several scary reports from others who had undergone cancer treatment and had horrible side effects. I didn't go back to the group for a long time.

I went ahead with the robotic surgery in October 2006, all the time focused on what might happen to my sexual potency. The first thing I did in the recovery room was to look under the blanket and check out my penis. It looked smaller to me, and I imagined that the end to my sex life as I had known it was just beginning. The surgeon was standing there and I said to him, "I thought you said my dick wasn't going to get any smaller." Later on, I heard that surgery leaves the dick a little bit smaller because they have to pull it in to re-attach the urethra to the bladder after the prostate gland is removed. This is actually not the case. A temporary shortening of the penis occurs because prostate surgery irritates the nerves that control erection. The nerves are not working then, depriving the penis of blood and oxygen. More permanent shortening of the penis (and eventual atrophy) happens only if, after surgery, nothing is done to regain blood flow and oxygen to stretch the penis. This is why most surgeons want their patients to masturbate and to take low doses of medications such as Viagra as soon as possible following prostate surgery.

After Surgery

I had a major complication after the surgery that had nothing to do with the robotic surgery itself. My stomach became extremely distended, and I was back in the hospital four days after the robotic surgery. My stomach was filling up, but the doctors couldn't find a problem. They discharged me, but I continued to get weaker and had more pain. After a week, my sister drove down to New York City and took me upstate where she lived. We drove straight to the local emergency room. I was admitted to intensive care with a diagnosis of renal failure. My kidneys were failing; everything was blocking up. The doctors told my sister I might not make it. The next step would be dialysis; however, just as they were arranging that, my kidneys slowly started to kick in. None of the doctors were able to give a definitive explanation for the renal failure. I don't think there was any connection between the robotic surgery and the renal failure. It was just a coincidence.

After a few weeks of recovery in that hospital and at

my sister's home, I returned to the upstate hospital to see an oncologist there. He thought I should have radiation to make sure all the cancer was gone. I came back to my home in New York City and went to an oncologist there who also recommended radiation. Because I wanted to be entirely cancer free, I took the same attitude I had when I chose robotic surgery: let's do it. In spring 2007 I had six weeks of external beam radiation, which wasn't as bad as I had imagined.

Depression and Loss of Erection

I was getting my strength and energy back after the radiation treatments; nonetheless, I sank into a deep depression. I was thankful that my PSA was now undetectable, and urinary incontinence wasn't that bad a problem. I did wet myself at night, however, because I take sleep medications that allow me sleep so soundly I miss the cues to urinate. To this day, it is still a trade-off: Do I get a good night's sleep and possibly wet myself, or forego the good sleep and wake up in a dry bed?

I was sinking deeper and deeper into a depression. For one thing, I could not work in my career because of the shoulder injury. I was now on disability. But, as odd as it may sound, the main thing that upset me was I couldn't get any erection at all. I felt I had lost my best friend. I tried Viagra and all the other drugs for treating erectile dysfunction (ED); nothing worked. Even though I couldn't get an erection, I still had pretty intense orgasms with a soft dick. That didn't matter: I wanted my hard dick back.

I then sought out a urologist who specialized in ED. He recommended penile injections, where the man injects himself at the base of the penis with a fluid that helps him get hard. This ended up failing because we couldn't regulate the dosage. It was either too little or too much. When it was too much, the shot did get me hard, but I would then stay hard for four hours. After the first thirty minutes of the erection, it became unbearably painful, and I could barely walk. I tried it several times and always ended up with a painful four-hour hard-on. Each time I said I'm not doing this again. But then I would, because I was desperate to get my dick back. After about eight attempts, because of the pain, I gave up trying the injections.

I was getting more and more depressed. I was frustrated and very sad. I cried a lot. I became overweight. Food was my only comfort. I couldn't stand looking at what I considered to be my mutilated body.

As a gay man, my preferred role in sex is to penetrate another man. Before the surgery, when I was topping somebody, it would make me feel like a man. I could step up to the plate with the best of them. It gave me such a high. My hard dick and I were very good friends. Now I felt like a eunuch.

It wasn't so much that I wanted to have sex with a guy as much as I wanted to feel powerful and manly, and to like my body again. Although I preferred being a top, during this period, I tried being a bottom. I was surprised to find out that bottoming wasn't as painful now as it was before the surgery. I guess with the prostate gland removed, there is more room.

When the injections failed, the ED specialist wanted me to try a medical vacuum pump. So we ordered it for $500, which my health insurance paid for. The thing—a huge cylinder— was just enormous. I tried it once, but it was just too much trouble. Two years after the surgery, nothing was working for me in terms of regaining sexual potency—not the Viagra, not the injections, not the vacuum pump. I was extremely frustrated.

I had heard about an operation for a penile implant, technically called an "inflatable penile prosthesis," from the New York oncologist who did my radiation. In this procedure, the surgeon inserts plastic tubes down the length of the penis, inserts a sack of fluid behind the pubic area, and inserts a "third ball" in the scrotum that contains a pump that the man uses to "inflate" and "deflate" the penis as needed. I wanted to have the penile implant, but the ED specialist didn't want me to do it yet. He recommended that I keep trying the injections and the pump. He believed that even if I was going to have the penile implant, my atrophied dick needed to be "stretched" more before they inserted the plastic tubes.

By this time, in 2008, I had returned to the Malecare group because I had gotten so depressed. One other group member was preparing to have the penile implant operation. About this time I learned about a surgeon at another hospital who was having success with the implants.

When the penile implant option came up, a cousin of mine could not imagine why I would do such a thing. It seemed extreme to her. She couldn't understand it; she felt it just wasn't necessary. But then something interesting happened. Shortly after she turned sixty, she developed breast cancer and was told she may need a mastectomy. As she goes through the agony of possibly losing her natural breasts, she has a better understanding of the sexual parts of the body being mutilated. It's really the same thing that both men and women go through when their sexuality is threatened. But I think it's worse for men because we don't get the same recognition of the loss of our sexuality. Prostate cancer causes more shame than breast cancer, I think.

The Penile Implant Surgery

In June 2009, I got my "inflatable penile prosthesis." People ask me if I was anxious about doing it, but I wasn't nervous at all. In fact, I was happy. I was about to get something I really needed. It felt like I was going in for a facelift. My dick was so shriveled at that point I felt they couldn't do any more damage to it.

Penile implant surgery is an outpatient procedure, and I was sent home with a lot of painkiller medication. My whole pubic area, penis, and scrotum were swollen enormously, and I couldn't go out in public without wearing a long shirt. The painkillers managed the pain, but without them, the pain was unremitting and constant. It took about two months to become completely pain free. My penis was very sensitive; I couldn't tolerate underwear or any clothing rubbing against it.

Two weeks after the surgery, I went back to the surgeon to try out the implant. The surgeon pressed my "third ball" for the first time, and my dick came to life! I was absolutely thrilled. I couldn't believe it. This thing seems to defy normal aging. I only need annual checkups now to show the surgeon that everything is working properly.

For a while, I had some difficulty locating the correct spot on the "third ball" in my scrotum to inflate the penis, but eventually I mastered it. The penis stays hard as long as I want, then I deflate it, by pressing a valve on the "third ball."

Compared to the dick I used to have, it's not the same. Before, when I used to get hard, the head of my dick would get really hot and engorged with blood. Because those tubes don't go all the way into the head of the penis, the head just doesn't get as hot and hard. I was also told that the head of my penis has some nerve damage. But I am not complaining.

I can feel the tubes very slightly inside my dick, but it's not a problem. There is no more atrophy of my dick! I am able to penetrate a man with about the same degree of hardness as before I had the prostate surgery.

There is one side effect from the penile implant that bothers some men, but I don't mind it. Your dick stays permanently semi-hard. For me, it's a reminder of my masculinity. I wear briefs or a jockstrap to contain my semi-erection. For guys who wear boxers, it might be a problem.

Physically and mentally, I am now a different person. I wholeheartedly recommend the penile implant procedure when everything else fails. The pain afterward was worth it. I feel like a new man. Sometimes I tell my sex partners about the implant. Some men are fascinated by it and want to see how it works. They think it's great. I only inflate my dick if I am going to penetrate someone.

There's one thing I'd like to tell other gay men facing prostate cancer. You need to know that if all else fails in terms of regaining your sexual potency after the surgery, the penile implant procedure is an option. I don't think the penile implant alterative is emphasized enough by doctors when discussing possible erectile dysfunction after cancer treatment. I think if I had known about it from the beginning, I would have been much less depressed and frustrated. If you do experience ED and all else fails, keeping the penile implant in the back of your mind can bring hope, and makes the recovery psychologically easier.

Coping with Advanced Prostate Cancer as a Gay Man

"Charles Godfry"

Initial Diagnosis and Treatment

I am a fifty-seven-year-old single gay man. I realized that I was gay at the age of fourteen. It took me another fourteen years but I finally came out at the age of twenty-eight. Prior to coming out to friends and a few people at work, I had had sex with only two people, both men. I had never kissed a man before that. I had kissed girls, but it was truly boring for me. My first year out was a wonderful blast of freedom. I had sex with about twelve to fifteen guys who I met through friends. Sometimes they were already friends who I had been too timid to approach. My circle of sexual partners was small, but it may have saved me from becoming HIV-positive as few of my friends or other people I had sex with ever developed it. I soon met someone, and we had an eight-year relationship, which was alternately wonderful and not so wonderful. I have not been in a relationship that lasted more than two months in the interim, but I did date. Mostly it was just sex. My favorite method of connecting for casual sex was the phone lines. I enjoyed hearing other men's fantasies and their voices while they described them. And so it went.

Then in November of 1998, at the age of forty-six, I had my first surgery ever; it was to repair a hernia. By January of 1999, I began experiencing trouble urinating but simply attributed it to the surgery. Finally, about a month later, I was referred to a urologist. Time and anxiety have clouded my memory, but I do recall that he checked my PSA level and revealed to me that it was thirty-two. The

271

gravity of that number was expressed by the fact that the doctor's eyes watered when he told me. My stomach turned, but I somehow remained calm on the outside. I asked what the next step would be. I was probably in shock. The following week I had a biopsy in which six samples were extracted from my prostate. Five or six of the specimens showed evidence of tumors. I had forgotten how rough this period had been for me until putting it down on paper. I can remember calling a friend who came and just sat with me silently in my apartment for the better part of ninety minutes. That helped make me feel safer and calmer. I should add that at this point I only told eight or ten friends about my having prostate cancer. I did not even tell my parents until five or six months later when the all the tests had been completed and clearly showed that the cancer had not metastasized. My father had gone through treatment for prostate cancer that was much less severe ten years earlier. We rarely spoke about it and never really sat down and discussed it.

I was referred to a cancer specialist at New York University Hospital during the winter of 1999; he put me through a number of tests: MRIs, CT scans, and so forth. They all showed that I had prostate cancer. Fortunately, the cancer had not spread outside the prostate gland. That was good news. But the fact that my PSA was so high indicated that the cancer was probably also in the tissue around the prostate. I was put on Casodex and then given a Lupron or Zoladex shot to reduce my PSA and shrink my prostate gland. Then I was scheduled for external beam radiation at NYU, starting in August. Although the treatment only lasted about eight weeks, it seemed like forever to get on with it. To top it all off, on Labor Day weekend, I developed a severe flu that lasted for two weeks and resulted in temperatures over 102, thus stopping the treatments for that period. My treatment ended up taking about eleven weeks to complete. I had to wait from about

April to August to begin my radiation treatment. I now wonder if that hiatus had anything to do with the cancer coming back about three years later, and if the delay in treatment caused my cancer to get out of control. I do remember being impatient that it took so long to get scheduled for radiation and worrying about my PSA increasing during that waiting period. But, then again, I thought I had been put on hormone suppressants, so why worry?

The shots and Casodex began in May and the radiation began in early August. In terms of the radiation treatment, the route to the hospital every day was complicated by the fact that I had to change subway trains several times to get there. I was usually scheduled for treatment in the early to mid-afternoon during or after lunch. I quickly had it all timed so that I could call the technicians from the office and find out if they were on schedule; there was a bar/restaurant about a block away from the hospital that had great food and where I could call again to see if I should hurry over or take my time or, depending on the radiation schedule go over immediately and then eat afterwards. I'd been given a very restricted list of non-fiber, non-oily, non-acid things I could eat. For the first two to three weeks, I ate normally and didn't have any reaction to the radiation; but that didn't last. I ate spaghetti with tomato sauce one evening and a side effect in the form of diarrhea became a harsh reality. Diarrhea hardly describes it. It was more like dysentery. Nothing would stay in my system once that began. A great way to lose weight was the only positive way to look at it. Tomato-based spaghetti sauce and all the rest were now off the diet, and it was really important that I stick to the restricted diet. Thankfully, I like asparagus and could tolerate beets. I also appreciate a baked potato and grilled chicken, and they were just fine then. The thing I really missed eating was a salad. Still, this was one of the periods when I felt most positive; despite the side effects, I felt confident that the procedure was being done for a purpose and that it would help me get rid of the cancer. I really felt good mentally and actually cheerful and optimistic. It was a rather (and this may sound strange) exhilarating challenge to get to and from my office to the radiation clinic in a timely fashion. Another side effect that got me was fatigue. I got up at normally at about 7:30 A.M. I would get tired and ready to leave the office and go straight home at 5:00 or 6:00 P.M. I went to bed at about 10:00 P.M. I became very relaxed about this routine, and although my work suffered, I didn't let it get me down mentally.

The treatment must have ended in late October. I soon found that my PSA had gone to zero. I was elated. Imagine the high that produced. I remained on Casodex for the next few years, but that was a minor inconvenience. The doctors had told me that the side effects of the hormone suppressants would fade in about three months. It ended up taking longer—until about August 2000. I really was patient about that and tried to explain to the few friends who knew about the diagnosis that putting on a porn video held little interest for me compared to The New Yorker magazine that was on my nightstand. During the initial hormone shots in 1999, I had hot flashes but no breast enlargement or weight gain. The hot flashes were pretty minor compared with what other men who have been on hormones have described to me.

I had a summer-share out on Long Island, where I was with a few friends and mostly new acquaintances. One friend who knew about the cancer, in spite of my wishes, told everyone in the house. I wondered why everyone suddenly got very comforting around me. That was just about the last time I confided in many people. Public discussion and gossip was just not what I wanted. Knowledge of the condition was kept to a few selected friends.

The Highs after Treatment

Then the sex drive returned. My first experience after the treatments was in August 2000 (it took that long), when I topped two partners in their bed. That worked for me. And that pattern, along with connecting by phone, which I much preferred to bars, became my routine. I met a fuck buddy in December who used to come over once every month or two. I had the best sex of my life with him. It was never personal with him and we were never seen out socially; he was one of three reasons I decided to take a share in a beach house on Fire Island in an area known as The Pines, which is a summer Mecca for gay men. One of the other reasons was a wonderful buddy that I met out on the beach on Long Island the summer before; and the third reason had to do with seeing the movie Long Time Companion again on cable. I liked the camaraderie depicted during scenes filmed there.

I took a half-share (rather than a quarter-share) to get the full experience. And I really did. I knew nothing about drugs; nothing up to that point. I took my first ecstasy (a popular disco-drug) before going to see Madonna at Madison Square Garden. There I was at the concert and the top of my head suddenly exploded. I felt fantastic. My friend and I went out bar hopping until about 3:00 A.M. on a school night. The social pattern in The Pines became Low Tea, High Tea, dinner and then The Pavilion to dance, which meant ecstasy. How can one explain to anyone who never went there what the old Pavilion dance club on Fire Island was like? It was grungy and falling down, loud and full of nooks and crannies around the edges for taking bumps of Ketamine ("Special K") and cocaine and crystal meth. My house in The Pines was a conglomerate of about sixteen guys who didn't really know each other and so there was no real schedule, and I didn't socialize with them except at the occasional dinner. I would go out with my friend from Long Island, who also took a half-share, and we soon made other new friends by July. Going out on both Friday and Saturday was the norm; Saturday until the Pavilion closed at 6:00 A.M., and then we would crash until noon. I could sleep well then, and the effect of the weekend only hit me on Tuesday evenings. I will never forget how good it felt to do ecstasy and "K" together. I had never felt that good since I was a little child, and the world was all cozy and safe with parents who adored me. There was a real sense of belonging. It wasn't really about sex. There was not that much for me that summer, and my fuck buddy and I would take the summer off during The Pines summer season. I had two friends now who would be on the dance floor with me, and as long as we could see each other and be just about an arm's length or two apart, it felt supportive and comfortable. I took a share in a new house for the next four years and I liked the arrangement of dinners and organization, although one of the house parents didn't really like my drug use. The really wonderful period lasted for three fabulous summers.

I also discovered other friends and other playgrounds in New York City. I went to the Roxy nightclub at least once a month from the fall to the spring. And I went to the Black Party and many other similar events. I learned how to smuggle in drugs effectively. Once I got caught with drugs going into a club a little early and they just took them away; they let me in the club and said not to get caught again in the next six months. Inside I saw my dealer and the same products that they took away. He knew who to pay off. Cash was all that was needed.

There were certain side effects I described which occur right away and are typical with radiation treatment, but suddenly new symptoms began to appear. I had no cum. That's part of the radiation treatment, and I knew that it was to be expected. I would feel like I was ejaculating but nothing came out and the feeling was not quite as intense as it had been before the cancer. I occasionally ejaculated blood, to the shock of a very patient partner. I also had a slow leak in my bladder. It gave me the chance of having a camera put up my urethra, and I could see the inside of my bladder. It eventually went away, but not before I pissed blood, occasionally clots of blood. None of this bothered me. I also passed blood in my stool during this period. I just got over it and kept the doctor informed because none of this really bothered me. I still had a sex drive and could get full erections and my PSA was still zero.

Then the Party Comes to an End

And then in the spring of 2003, the PSA started to climb again at about a point a month. My first urologist seemed dismissive and said that there "wasn't anything" he could do for me. It seemed like a kiss-off. I went to Columbia Presbyterian Hospital to try cryogenic therapy, which involves freezing the prostate to get all the cancer. The risk of impotence with this treatment is high, and so I managed to make a mental list of all the people I wanted to have sex with before I underwent treatment, and my luck wasn't bad that summer. I had the cryosurgery in September 2003. And yes, I was impotent as a result. What had always been easy, like masturbation, wasn't as easy anymore. I had commonly had safe sex with one to five partners in a week and had about one to three orgasms a day before the procedure. It was the rudest of awakenings.

Penile implants seemed invasive and absurd to me. Injections to get my penis hard seemed equally absurd. I tried that about two times and could just imagine excusing myself with an anonymous sex partner to run into the bathroom for a quick injection. This also says a lot about my impatience with other people. I assumed other people would be as coldly sexual as I probably was before. It also says a lot about not investing any time in developing any kind of real relationship, which I now regret.

The PSA ironically began to climb at an even quicker rate: two points a month. Obviously, the cancer was somewhere outside the prostate itself and probably in the adjacent tissue or (hopefully not) elsewhere. I was now referred to an oncologist, which made me nervous and a bit scared and feeling like this was a last ditch effort. The solution for this rise in PSA was alternating hormone-suppressing shots of Lupron and Zoladex with periods of being off the suppressants. I began to develop tenderness in my pecs and then it would go away. My new doctor said that I probably experienced that in puberty. I didn't know what he was talking about. This treatment worked for about three years. In the meantime, my sex life was now just about nil as I bounced back and forth from occasional desire to brief spurts of lust. And depression began to occur.

Depression is looking in a closet full of clean shirts in the morning and finding that they all look ugly and that it takes you about a half an hour to choose one; it's not wanting to get up in the morning. I was never a morning person, but this was something else. The psychiatrist I went to said that I was manic-depressive. I just felt depressive depressive. Trazodone and other anti-depressants did nothing for me. Wellbutrin helped to some degree. Well, maybe I was always a manic depressive. I can stand back and realize that now. Being a person who doesn't have a sex drive gives one a lot of time to think about past feelings and ponder them. I was always someone who let others suggest things to do. I think that began when I discovered I was gay. As I hid my knowledge of this, it must have made me more and more repressed and perhaps depressed.

Then in 2007, my oncologist came in and muttered something about metastasis. I asked him to speak up. The cancer had spread to the lymph nodes in an area under my heart. This pains me just to write it. I completely deny this to myself every day by putting it out of my mind, as I am doing again right now. Since that time, I have been on Lupron constantly. The PSA, however, continued to rise. The oncologist took me off Casodex and my PSA dropped dramatically to the low digits. And then it began to rise again in late 2008. The solution for this was to go on an anti-fungal drug called Ketaconazole. Three tablets a day didn't have any affect. Two pills three times a day along with hydrocortisone did have an effect and the PSA has continued to go down to 0.4 from 0.9. I feel great about that.

One of the main things about this depression is not having anything to look forward to and often feeling like it's difficult to be cheerful. My friends often tell me to smile. Hours of not being able to do what one is supposed to be doing is another symptom. One thing that was noticeable beginning about four years ago was a lack of pleasure in listening to music at home, especially rock music. I never realized how much the enjoyment of it has to do with testosterone. That's a drug that really makes someone appreciate a beat. Somehow now the new Pavilion and the Roxy (I was there on closing night) didn't hold any interest. I had sex with one person in the last year or two. I was high from that for weeks. I had seen him the night before and been instantly attracted. It turned out he felt the same about me and we finally sat side-by-side at the bar the next night when he passed me a charming note and grabbed my crotch. One effect of the radiation is that one can have incontinence, i.e., wet crotch, especially when alcohol is involved. For once, luckily it was dry. And we were both pretty ripped. We began to make out and when he grabbed my crotch I said that he wouldn't find much there. He said, "Prostate cancer?" "Yes," I replied. "Oh, my dad had that," he said, and just continued. We went back to his place. I went down on him (or at least got on my knees) and he valiantly tried to suck me off: a losing proposition for both of us. I could not care less if I had an orgasm, but I do care about not getting an erection. But at least the thrill was there. It makes me wonder if I care about anything except sex.

Where am I now? I do look forward to dating and should look forward to it. Meaning really taking the time to get to know someone and listen to him. And I have to grow up, even though the lack of testosterone seems to make life depressing. But that encounter with the guy whose father had prostate cancer gave me some hope that I can have sensual and emotional connections in the future.

Right now I find that I really have to force myself do things, and it'll have to be that way for now. I am depressed. I don't expect to have a sex life with the almost-total chemical castration that has occurred with the injections and Ketaconazole. Photographs of beautiful men used to be a turn on, but now that isn't the case. My tastes are really particular: men with silver hair, extremely handsome young men, and men that I really respect are a turn on. It's just that it's going to be next to impossible to act or follow through on any attraction because the drive just isn't there without testosterone. It's hard to explain to someone who still has a sex drive. The drive has turned to food and drink. I really feel good when I am drinking and so look forward to the evenings when I can fill those desires, which are obviously a replacement for sex. The drinking is a bit excessive, although I do seem to know my limits. I look forward to eating and am particular about food now in a way that I wasn't before.

There are times when I am reminded of the old desires and they seem like distant memories and it seems that it's probably the way someone feels at eighty. Or at least I feel that way most of the time in spite of looking relatively fit for my age. All in all, I feel that I just have to take it a day at a time and try to keep as positive an attitude as possible. Most importantly, I still feel that I will stay healthy. It makes me happy to say that the period of partying in The Pines produced a number of wonderful friendships, and I keep up with many of those friends on a regular basis. The whole experience gave me an opening to a whole new group of people who I never would have met otherwise. Whenever I am down, I just think of that.

GLOSSARY

ABIRATERONE ACETATE: A new hormone therapy that blocks the enzyme that facilitates the production of testosterone both in the testes and in other testosterone-producing tissues in the body. It is still in early clinical trial stages for men with advanced prostate cancer.

ABLATION: The removal or excision of a body part or the destruction of its function.

ACTIVE SURVEILLANCE: An option for men with low-grade, early-stage cancers to forego invasive procedures; and instead, to have regular checkups to monitor their PSA score, have DREs, and typically have annual biopsies. (See WATCHFUL WAITING.)

ADENOCARCINOMA: A form of cancer that develops from malignant abnormality in cells lining a glandular organ; almost all prostate cancers are of this variety.

ADJUVANT THERAPY: Treatment used in addition to the main treatment, such as radiation therapy and hormonal therapy, which are often used as adjuvant treatments following a radical prostatectomy.

ANDROGEN: Any male sex hormone, the major one being testosterone.

ANTIANDROGENS: Drugs that block or interfere with the body's ability to use androgens at the cellular receptor sites. Antiandrogens used to treat prostate cancer include the brand names Eulexin, Casodex, and Nilandron.

ANTICHOLINERGIC: A drug that may block the parasympathetic nerves, such as blocking the bladder and genitalia. It may be used to treat urinary incontinence among other conditions.

BENIGN PROSTATIC HYPERPLASIA (BPH): Non-cancerous enlargement of the prostate that may restrict urine flow.

BIOPSY: A procedure in which the physician places a narrow needle through the wall of the rectum into the prostate in order to obtain samples of tissue to ascertain if cancer is present. This is done with the guidance of ultrasound.

BRACHYTHERAPY: A form of radiation therapy in which radioactive seeds are implanted in order to kill surrounding tissue. It is also called interstitial radiation therapy or SEED IMPLANTATION (SI).

CAPSULE: The fibrous outer lining of cells around an organ such as the prostate.

CARCINOMA: A form of cancer that originates in tissues that line or cover a particular organ.

CATHETER (URINARY): A thin, flexible tube through which fluids enter or leave the body. It is common for prostate cancer patients to have a transurethral catheter (Foley) in order to drain urine for time after certain treatments.

CAVERJECT: A brand name of Alprostadil, which is a drug used to treat erectile dysfunction (ED). It is injected directly into the penis; it produces an erection by relaxing the trabecular smooth muscle and by dilating the cavernosal arteries localized in the penis. See MUSE.

CLIMACTURIA: The inadvertent loss of urine at orgasm, often following radical prostatectomy.

COMBINED HORMONAL TREATMENT (CHT): The blocking of the production of androgen (prostate testosterone) through surgical or chemical castration plus the use of anti-androgen hormone therapy. Also called total hormonal ablation, total androgen blockade, or total androgen ablation.

CONFORMAL RADIATION THERAPY (CRT): Planning and delivery techniques designed to focus radiation on the areas of the prostate and surrounding tissue that need treatment while protecting areas which do not need treatment. 3-D CONFORMAL therapy (3-D CRT) is a sophisticated form of this method.

CRYOSURGERY: Freezing of the prostate transperineally in order to kill the tissue, including cancerous tissue, by using liquid nitrogen probes guided by transrectal ultrasound imaging of the prostate. (Also called CRYOABLATION.)

DIGITAL RECTAL EXAMINATION (DRE): The physician's use of a lubricated gloved finger inserted into the rectum in order to feel for abnormalities of the prostate and rectum.

DISSEMINATED DISEASE: A disease that is widespread.

DOWNSIZING: The use of hormonal or other treatment modalities to reduce the volume of prostate cancer in and/or around the prostate prior to other curative treatment.

DYSURIA: Painful or burning urination.

ENDORECTAL ULTRASOUND: A procedure in which a probe that sends out high-energy sound waves is inserted into the rectum to seek out abnormalities in the rectum or surrounding areas, particularly the prostate gland. (Also called ERUS, TRANSRECTAL ULTRASOUND, and TRUS.)

EXTERNAL BEAM RADIATION (EBRT): A form of radiation therapy in which the radiation is delivered by a machine focused on the area affected by the cancer. (It is also called EXTERNAL RADIATION THERAPY.)

FLOMAX (Tamsulosin): A drug used to relax the prostate and bladder neck to improve urine flow.

FOLEY TRACTION: A technique used in prostatectomies. During surgery a urinary catheter is placed in the urethra and tension is applied. This pulls the inflated bladder of the Foley catheter against the base of the bladder, creating some control of bleeding. It unfortunately also has the effect of placing the neurovascular bundle controlling erections, abutting the prostate, under tension as well. (See CATHETER.)

FREE-PSA: This indicates how much PSA circulates unbound in the blood and how much is bound together with other blood proteins; the percentage of free-PSA to total-PSA. A low percent of free-PSA (25% or less) suggests that a prostate cancer is more likely to be present. It is a useful screening device when PSA values are above normal but less than 10. (It is also called PSA-II.)

GLEASON SCORE: A method of classifying prostate cancer cells on a scale from 2 to 10. The higher the number, the more undifferentiated the cells, and the faster the cancer is likely to grow. A ranking of 1-5 is assigned to the two most predominant patterns of differentiation present in the tissue sample examined. These numbers are added together to yield a total Gleason score. Scores of 2-4 indicate well-differentiated cells; 5-6 indicates tumors with cells beginning to scatter; and scores of 7-10 indicate poorly differentiated cells.

HAART: An acronym for "Highly-Active Antiretroviral Therapy" used in the treatment of HIV.

HORMONE THERAPY: The use of medication or surgery to interfere with hormone production or action. Because prostate cancer is usually dependent on male hormones to grow, hormonal therapy is used to block or lower testosterone.

HIGH DOSE RATE (HDR): The temporary implanting of radioactive seeds into the prostate, followed by external beam radiation (EBRT).

HYPOGONADAL: A medical term for decreased functional activity of the testicles involving reduced levels of testosterone.

IMPOTENCE: The inability to have or to maintain an erection; erectile dysfunction (ED).

INTENSITY-MODULATED RADIATION THERAPY (IMRT): A computer-generated program that pinpoints the cancer for radiation treatment.

INCONTINENCE: The loss of urinary control.

ISOFLAVONES: A class of anti-oxidant organic

compounds that may be antagonistic to breast and prostate cancer.

KEGEL EXERCISES: Exercises designed to improve the strength of the muscles controlling urination.

KETOCONAZOLE: A synthetic antifungal agent which, when given in high doses, has testosterone lowering effects by blocking various endocrine pathways. It is a form of androgen deprivation therapy. Common brand names are Nizoral, Extina, Xolegel, and Kuric.

LAPAROSCOPY: A technique in which the surgeon can observe the internal organs by inserting a tube with optic capacity into small surgical incisions in the body.

LUTEINIZING HORMONE RELEASING HORMONE (LHRH): A chemical that blocks the production of testosterone by the testes that may be used as part of hormone therapy of prostate cancer. Lupron and Zoladex are common brand names.

LYCOPENE: An antioxidant found in tomatoes, raspberries, and watermelon; laboratory studies have indicated that it may have a beneficial effect against prostate cancer. It is available as a dietary supplement.

MUSE: A brand name for a form of Alprostadil in the form of a suppository inserted into the urethra to treat erectile dysfunction. (See CAVERJECT.)

NADIR: The lowest point reached, for example, in a series of PSA values following radiation.

NERVE-SPARING: A term used to describe a type of prostatectomy in which the surgeon saves the nerves that affect sexual functioning.

NOCTURIA: The need to urinate frequently at night. Sometimes it is called NYCTURIA.

NOMOGRAM: A chart representing varying numerical relationships.

ONCOLOGIST: A physician specializing in the treatment of cancer.

ORCHIECTOMY: The surgical removal of the testicles; castration.

PALLIATION: The partial treating of a disease as far as possible, but not completely; often to relieve pain, symptoms, or the stress of a serious illness.

PARTIN TABLES: These are tables that use PSA values, Gleason score, and clinical stage of prostate cancer to predict the likelihood of organ confinement, as well as capsule, seminal-vesicle, and lymph node involvement.

PARTIN II TABLES: These are tables that use PSA growth rate after prostatectomy to distinguish local recurrence from distant metastasis.

PC SPES: The brand name for a dietary supplement that is used to lower PSA in prostate cancer; it is no longer available. PC Plus appears to be a new generation of this herbal supplement. (See SAW PALMETTO.)

PERINEAL PROSTATECTOMY: An operation to remove the prostate gland via an incision made between the anus and the scrotum (The area called the PERINEUM.)

PIN CELLS: (See PROSTATIC INTRAEPITHELIAL NEOPLASIA.)

PLETHYSMOGRAPHY: The use of an instrument to measure changes in volume within an organ or the whole body.

PROSTATIC INTRAEPITHELIAL NEOPLASIA (PIN): A pathologically identifiable condition thought to be a possible precursor of prostate cancer. (It is also known as DYSPLASIA.)

PROSTATE: The walnut-sized gland in the male reproductive system that surrounds the urethra and is immediately below the bladder. Its primary function is to supply fluid for semen to transport sperm during ejaculation.

PROSTATECTOMY: The surgical removal of part or all of the prostate gland.

PROSTATE-SPECIFIC ANTIGEN (PSA): A protein secreted by the prostate gland that is used to detect potential problems in the prostate; it is also used to follow the progress of prostate cancer therapy. Elevated levels may indicate an abnormal condition, which may be malignant or benign.

PROSTATITIS: Inflammation of the prostate. It is not cancer.

PROTON BEAM THERAPY (PBT): A form of radiation that uses protons to treat cancer tumors; the proton beam is focused on the cancer site. Protons are sub-particles of an atom that are absorbed by the tumor. (It is also called PROTON BEAM RADIATION.)

PROVENGE (Sipuleucel-T): An immunotherapy for the treatment of minimally or non-symptomatic hormone refractory advanced prostate cancer that has recently been approved by the FDA.

PSA VELOCITY (PSAV): The rate at which PSA values increase. A higher PSAV indicates a greater likelihood of cancer being present.

QUALITY-OF-LIFE (QOL): An evaluation of health status relative to a patient's age, expectations, and physical and mental capacities.

RADIATION ONCOLOGIST: A physician specializing in the treatment of cancers with the use of various types of radiation.

RADIATION THERAPY (RT): The use of radiation to destroy malignant cells and tissues.

RADICAL PROSTATECTOMY (RP): Surgery to remove the entire prostate gland, the seminal vesicles, and nearby tissue.

RETROPUBIC PROSTATECTOMY: The surgical removal of the prostate through a vertical incision in the abdomen.

SAW PALMETTO: One of the eight herbs that comprise PC SPES. It decreases the bioavailability of testosterone in laboratory studies.

STAGE: A term used to define the size and extent of a cancer. For example, Stage T1c: Tumor cannot be felt on digital rectal exam, but only through needle biopsy. Stage T2a: Tumor is confined within the prostate gland and is minimally detected in one half lobe of the prostate or less.

TRANSPERINEAL: Through the perineum.

TRANSRECTAL: Through the rectum.

TRANSURETHRAL RESECTION OF THE PROSTATE (TURP): A surgical procedure to remove prostate tissue obstructing the urethra and thus urine flow. It is sometimes used to determine Gleason score.

URETHRITUS: Inflammation of the urethra.

URINARY SLING: A mesh strip that is surgical placed to support the urethra during straining movements like laughing, coughing, jumping, and so forth, thus reducing urinary leakage.

WATCHFUL WAITING (WW): The active observation and regular monitoring of a man with prostate cancer without actual treatment. (Also called EXPECTANT MANAGEMENT and/or ACTIVE SURVEILLANCE.)

ZYFLAMEND: An herbal supplement consisting of ten herbs, including basil, turmeric, ginger, green tea, rosemary, and other Chinese herbs. It is reported to have anti-inflammatory and anti-aging properties. Small and inconclusive studies suggest it may inhibit the proliferation of human prostate cancer cells.

References Listed According to Essay

References re: *Gay Men's Knowledge of Prostate Caner*

Agho, A. O., & Lewis, M. A. (2001). Correlates of actual and perceived knowledge of prostate cancer among African-Americans. *Cancer Nursing*, 24, 165-171.

Albarran, J. W., & Salmon, D. (2000). Lesbian, gay and bisexual experiences within critical care nursing, 1988-1998: A survey of the literature. *International Journal of Nursing Studies*, 37, 445-455.

Allen, J. D., Kennedy, M., Wilson-Glover, A., & Gilligan, T. D. (2007). African-American men's perceptions about prostate cancer: Implications for designing educational interventions. *Social Science and Medicine*, 64, 2189-2200.

Allensworth-Davies, D., & Clark, J. (2008, May). *Diagnosis and treatment of localized prostate cancer: The gay male experience*. Presented at the Midcontinent and Eastern Region Joint Conference, Society for the Scientific Study of Sexuality, Cleveland, OH.

American Cancer Society. (2009). *Cancer facts & figures 2009*. Atlanta, GA: American Cancer Society.

Asencio, M., Blank, T., Descartes, L., & Crawfoed, A. (*2009*). The prospect of cancer: A challenge for gay men's sexualities as they age. *Sexuality Research and Social Policy*, 6 (4), 38-51.

Blank, T. O. (*In press*). Cancer from both sides now: Combining personal and research perspectives on survivorship. *Journal of General Internal Medicine*, DOI 10.1007/s11606-009-1018-5.

Blank, T. O., Asencio, M., Descartes, L., & Griggs, J. (2009). Aging, health, and GLBTQ family and community life. *Journal of GLBT Family Studies*, 5, 9-34.

Bonvicini, K. A., & Perlin, M. J. (2003). The same but different: Clinician patient communication with gay and lesbian patients. *Patient Education and Counseling*, 51, 115-122.

Chan, E. C. Y., Vernon, S. W., O'Donnell, F. T., Ahn, C., Greisinger, A., & Aga, D. W. (2003). Informed consent for cancer screening with prostate-specific antigen: How well are men getting the message? *American Journal of Public Health*, 93, 779-785.

Chapple, A., & Ziebland, S. (2002). Prostate cancer: Embodied experience and perceptions of masculinity. *Sociology of Health and Illness*, 24, 820-841.

Deibert, C. M., Maliski, S., Kwan, L., Fink, A., Connor, S. E. & Litwin, M. S. (2007). Prostate cancer knowledge among low income minority men. *The Journal of Urology*, 177, 1851-1855.

Fergus, K. D., Gray, R. E., & Fitch, M. I. (2002). Sexual dysfunction and the preservation of manhood: Experience of men with prostate cancer. *Journal of Health Psychology*, 7, 303-316.

Filiault, S. M., Drummond, M. J. N., & Smith, J. A. (2008). Gay men and prostate cancer: Voicing the concerns of a hidden population. *Journal of Men's Health*, 5, 327-332.

Forrester-Anderson, I. T. (2005). Prostate cancer screening perceptions, knowledge, and behaviors among African-American men: Focus group findings. *Journal of Health care for the Poor and Underserved*, 16 (Suppl. A), 22-30.

Gay and Lesbian Medical Association. (2001). Healthy People 2010 companion document for lesbian, gay, bisexual, and transgender (LGBT) health. Retrieved from http://glma.org/policy/hp2010/.

Goldstone, S. E. (2005). The ups and downs of gay sex after prostate cancer treatment. In G. Perlman & J. Drescher (Eds.), *A Gay Man's Guide to Prostate Cancer* (pp. 43-55). New York: Haworth.

Gotay, C. C., Holup, J. L., & Muraoka, M. Y. (2002). Challenges of prostate cancer: A major men's health issue. *International Journal of Men's Health*, 1, 59-72.

Gray, R. E., Fitch, M. I., Fergus, K. D., Mykhalovskiy, E. & Church, K. (2002). Hegemonic masculinity and the experience of prostate cancer: A narrative approach. *Journal of Aging and Identity*, 7, 43-62.

Grunfeld, E. (2005). Cancer survivorship: A challenge for primary care physicians. *British Journal of General Practice*, 55, 741-742.

Hersom, J. W., Coon, D. W., Hart, S. L., & Latini, D. M. (2009, April). Quality-of-life for gay men treated for localized prostate cancer: Preliminary results from a web-based study. Presented at Society of Behavioral Medicine, Montreal, Quebec.

Heslin, K. C., Gore, J. L., King, W. D., & Fox, S. A. (2008). Sexual orientation and testing for prostate and colorectal cancers among men in California. *Medical Care*, 46, 1240-1248.

Kelly, D. (2009). Changed men: The embodied impact of prostate cancer. *Qualitative Health Research*, 19, 151-163.

Kilbridge, K. L., Fraser, G., Krahn, M., Nelson, E. M., Conaway, M., Bashore, R., et al. (2009). Lack of comprehension of common prostate cancer terms in an underserved population. *Journal of Clinical Oncology*, 27: 2015-2021. DOI: 10.1200/JCO.2008.17.368.

Kitzinger, J. (2006). Focus groups. In: (eds.) Pope, C., & Mays, N. *Qualitative Research in Health Care*, 3rd Ed. Malden, MA: Blackwell Publishing, pp. 21-31.

Litwin, M. S., Melmed, G. Y, & Nakazon, T. (2001). Life after radical prostatectomy: A longitudinal study. *Journal of Urology*, 166, 587-592.

Maliski, S. L., Connor, S., Fink, A., & Litwin, M. S. (2006). Information desired and acquired by men with prostate cancer: Data from ethic focus groups. *Health Education and Behavior*, 33, 393-409.

Marks, S. (2003). *Prostate and Cancer: A Family Guide to Diagnosis, Treatment, and Survival*. New York: Perseus.

McFall, S. L., Ureda, J., Byrd, T. L., Valdes, A., Morales, V. A., Scott, V. D., et al. (2009). What is needed for informed decisions about prostate cancer screening: Perspectives of African-American and Hispanic men. *Health Education Research*, 24, 280-291.

McGovern, R. J., Heyman, E. N., & Resnick, M. I. (2002). An examination of coping style and quality-of-life of cancer patients who attend a prostate cancer support group. *Journal of Psychosocial Oncology*, 20, 57-68.

Meade, C. D., Calvo, A., Rivera, M. A., & Baer, R. D. (2003). Focus groups in the design of prostate cancer screening information for Hispanic farm workers and African-American men. *Oncology Nursing Forum*, 30, 967-975.

Miksad, R. A., Bubley, G., Church, P., Sanda, M., Rofsky, N., Irving, K. et al. (2006). Prostate cancer in a transgender woman 41 years after initiation of feminization. *Journal of the American Medical Association*, 296, 2316-2317.

Newman, P. A., Roberts, K. J., Masongsong, E., & Wiley, D. J. (2008). Anal cancer screening: Barriers and facilitators among ethnically diverse gay, bisexual, transgender, and other men who have sex with men. *Journal of Gay and Lesbian Social Services*, 20, 328-353.

Oliffe, J. (2005). Constructions of masculinity following prostatectomy-induced impotence. *Social Science and Medicine*, 60, 2249-2259.

Oliffe, J. (2006). Embodied masculinity and androgen deprivation therapy. *Sociology of Health and Illness*, 28, 410-432.

Perlman, G., & Drescher, J. (2005). *A Gay Man's Guide to Prostate Cancer*. New York: Haworth.

Pugh, S. (2005). Assessing the cultural needs of older lesbians and gay men: Implications for practice. *Practice*, 17, 207-218.

Quek, M.L., & Penson, D.F. (2005). Quality-of-life in patients with localized prostate cancer. *Urological Oncology*, 23, 208-215.

Ramchand, R., & Fox, C. (2007). Access to optimal care among gay and bisexual men: Identifying barriers and promoting culturally competent care. In R. J. Wolitski, R. Stall, & R. O. Valdiserri (Eds.), *Unequal opportunity: Health disparities affecting gay and bisexual men in the United States* (pp. 355-378). New York: Oxford University Press.

Santillo, V. M., & Lowe, F. C. (2005). Prostate cancer and the gay male. *Journal of Gay & Lesbian Mental Health*, 9, 9-27.

Steele, C. B., Miller, D. S., Maylahn, C., Uhler, R. J., & Baker, C. T. (2000). Knowledge, attitudes, and screening practices among older men regarding prostate cancer. *American Journal of Public Health*, 90, 1595-1600.

Strong, B., Devault, C., Sayad, B. W., & Yarber, W. L. (Eds.). (2008). *Human Sexuality: Diversity in Contemporary America* (6th ed.). New York: McGraw-Hill.

Thaxton, L., Emshoff, J. G., & Guessous, O. (2005). Prostate cancer support groups. *Journal of Psycho-social Oncology*, 23, 25-40.

Thurman, N, Ragin, C., Heron, D. E., Alford, R. J., Andraos-Selim, C., Bondzi, C., et al. (2009). Comparison of knowledge and attitudes toward cancer among African-Americans. *Infectious Agents and Cancer*, 4 (Suppl. 1), S1-S15.

Trettin, S., Moses-Kolko, E.L, & Wisner, K.L. (2006).

Lesbian perinatal depression and the heterosexism that affects knowledge about this minority population. *Archives of Women's Mental Health*, 9, 67-73.

Wilkinson, S., List, M., Sinner, M., Dai, L., & Chodak, G. (2003). Educating African-American men about prostate cancer: Impact on awareness and knowledge. *Urology*, 61, 308-313.

References re: Quality-of-life and Cancer Control after Prostate Cancer

American Cancer Society (2009), *Cancer Facts & Figures 2009*.

Bella, A., & Lue, T. (2009). Optimizing sexual function outcomes after radical prostatectomy. *Can Urol Assoc J*, 3, 49.

Cooperberg, M., Lubeck, D., Meng, M., Mehta, S., & Carroll, P. (2004). The changing face of low-risk prostate cancer: Trends in clinical presentation and primary management. *J Clin Oncol*, 22, 2141-2149.

Eastham, J., Scardino, P., & Kattan, M. (2008). Predicting an optimal outcome after radical prostatectomy: The trifecta nomogram. *J Urol*, 179, 2207-2211.

Fowler, F., Collins, M., Albertsen, P., Zietman, A., Elliott, D., & Barry, M. (2000). Comparison of recommendations by urologists and radiation oncologists for treatment of clinically localized prostate cancer. *JAMA*, 283, 3217-3222.

Garcia, F., & Brock, G. (2010). Current state of penile rehabilitation after radical prostatectomy. *Curr Opin Urol*, 20, In Press.

Gore, J., Kwan, L., Lee, S., Reiter, R., & Litwin, M. (2009). Survivorship beyond convalescence: 48-month quality-of-life outcomes after treatment for localized prostate cancer. *J Natl Cancer Inst*, 101, 888-892.

Hu, J., Gu, X., Lipsitz, S., Barry, M., D'Amico, A., Weinberg, A., & Keating, N. (2009). Comparative effectiveness of minimally invasive vs. open radical prostatectomy. *JAMA*, 302, 1557-1564.

Kumar, A., Litt, E., Ballert, K., & Nitti, V. (2009). Artificial urinary sphincter vs. male sling for post-prostatectomy incontinence–what do patients choose? *J Urol*, 181, 1231-1235.

Lu-Yao, G, & Yao, S. (1997). Population-based study of long-term survival in patients with clinically localized prostate cancer. *Lancet*, 349, 906-910.

Masterson, T., Serio, A., Mulhall, J., Vickers, A., & Eastham, J. (2008). Modified technique for neurovascular bundle preservation during radical prostatectomy: Association between technique and recovery of erectile function. *BJU Int*, 101, 1217-1222.

Montorsi, F., Guazzoni, G., Strambi, L., Da Pozzo, F., Nava, L., Barbieri, L., Rigatti, P., Pizzini, G., & Miani, A. (1997). Recovery of spontaneous erectile function after nerve-sparing radical retropubic prostatectomy with and without early intracavernous injections of alprostadil: Results of a prospective, randomized trial. *J Urol*, 158, 1408-1410.

Montorsi, F., Brock, G., Lee, J., Shapiro, J., Van Poppel, H., Graefen, M., & Stief, C. (2008). Effect of nightly vs. on-demand vardenafil on recovery of erectile function in men following bilateral nerve-sparing radical prostatectomy. *Eur Urol*, 54, 924-931.

Mulhall, J., Land, S., Parker, M., Waters, W., & Flanigan, R. (2005). The use of an erectogenic pharmacotherapy regimen following radical prostatectomy improves recovery of spontaneous erectile function. *J Sex Med*, 2, 532-542.

Mulhall, J., & Morgentaler, A. (2007). Penile rehabilitation should become the norm for radical prostatectomy patients. *J Sex Med*, 4, 538-543.

Mulhall, J. (2009). Does on-demand vardenafil improve erectile function recovery after radical prostatectomy? *Nat Clin Pract Urol*, 6, 14-15.

Padma-Nathan, H., McCullough, A., Levine, L., Lipshultz, L., Siegel, R., Montorsi, F., Giuliano, F., & Brock, G. (2008). Randomized, double-blind, placebo-controlled study of postoperative nightly sildenafil citrate for the prevention of erectile dysfunction after bilateral nerve-sparing radical prostatectomy. *Int J Impot Res*, 20, 479-486.

Pisters, L. (2010). Cryotherapy for prostate cancer: ready for prime time? *Curr Opin Urol*, 20, Epub (In Press).

Sanda, M., Dunn, R., Michalski, J., Sandler, H., Northouse, L., Hembroff, L., Lin, X., Greenfield, T., Litwin, M., Saigal, C., Mahadevan, A., Klein, E., Kibel, A., Pisters, L., Kuban, D., Kaplan, I., Wood, D., Ciezki, J., Shah, N., & Wei, J. (2008). Quality-of-life and satisfaction with outcome among prostate-cancer survivors. *N Engl J Med*, 358, 1250-1261.

Shikanov, S., Zorn, K., Zagaja, G., & Shalhav, A. (2009). Trifecta outcomes after robotic-assisted laparoscopic prostatectomy. *Urology*, 74, 619-625.

Walsh, P., Lepor, H., & Eggleston, J. (1983). Radical prostatectomy with preservation of sexual function: Anatomical and pathological considerations. *Prostate*, 4,

473-485.

Wilt, T., Brawer, M., Barry, M., Jones, K., Kwon, Y., Gingrich, J., Aronson, W., Nsouli, I., Iyer, P., Cartagena, R., Snider, G., Roehrborn, C., & Fox, S. (2009). The prostate cancer intervention vs. observation trial: VA/NCI/AHRQ cooperative studies program #407 (PIVOT): Design and baseline results of a randomized controlled trial comparing radical prostatectomy to watchful waiting for men with clinically localized prostate cancer. *Contemp Clin Trials*, 30, 81-87.

References re: Prostate Cancer and Sexual Dysfunction in Gay Men

American Cancer Society (2009). How Many Men Get Prostate Cancer? http://www.cancer.org/docroot/CRI/content/CRI 2 2 1X How many men get prostate cancer 36.asp Updated: 08/21/2009, Accessed: 11/15/2009

Barnas, J. L., Pierpaoli, S., Ladd, P., Valenzuela, R., Aviv, N., Parker, M., Waters, W. B., Flanigan, R. C. and Mulhall, J. P. (2004). The prevalence and nature of orgasmic dysfunction after radical prostatectomy. *BJU Int, 94, 603-5.*

Blank, T. O. (2005). Gay men and prostate cancer: Invisible diversity. *J Clin Oncol, 23, 2593-6.*

De la Peyronie, F. (1743). Sur quelques obstacles qui s'opposent a` l'e´jaculation naturelle de la semence. *Mem Acad Roy Chir, 1, 425-434.*

Haliloglu, A., Baltaci, S. and Yaman, O. (2007). Penile length changes in men treated with androgen suppression plus radiation therapy for local or locally advanced prostate cancer. *J Urol, 177, 128-30.*

Huggins, C. and Hodges, C. V. (1941). The effect of castration, of estrogen and of androgen injection on serum phosphatases in metastatic carcinoma of the prostate. *Cancer Res, 1, 293-297.*

Jemal, A., Siegel, R., Ward, E., Hao, Y., Xu, J. and Thun, M. J. (2009). Cancer statistics, 2009. *CA Cancer J Clin, 59,*

225-49.

Levin, R. J. (2009). Revisiting post-ejaculation refractory time--what we know and what we do not know in males and in females. *J Sex Med, 6, 2376-89.*

Lue, T. F. (2000). Erectile dysfunction. *N Engl J Med, 342, 1802-13.*

Moreno, S. A. and Morgentaler, A. (2009). Testosterone deficiency and Peyronie's disease: Pilot data suggesting a significant relationship. *J Sex Med, 6, 1729-35.*

Morgentaler, A. (2009). Testosterone therapy in men with prostate cancer: Scientific and ethical considerations. *J Urol, 181, 972-9.*

Mulhall, J. P. (2008). Penile rehabilitation following radical prostatectomy. *Curr Opin Urol, 18, 613-20.*

Phan, J., Swanson, D. A., Levy, L. B., Kudchadker, R. J., Bruno, T. L. and Frank, S. J. (2009). Late rectal complications after prostate brachytherapy for localized prostate cancer: *Incidence and management. Cancer, 115, 1827-39.*

Sanda, M. G., Dunn, R. L., Michalski, J., Sandler, H. M., Northouse, L., Hembroff, L., Lin, X., Greenfield, T. K., Litwin, M. S., Saigal, C. S., Mahadevan, A., Klein, E., Kibel, A., Pisters, L. L., Kuban, D., Kaplan, I., Wood, D., Ciezki, J., Shah, N. and Wei, J. T. (2008). Quality-of-life and satisfaction with outcome among prostate-cancer survivors. *N Engl J Med, 358, 1250-61.*

Sanderson, K. M., Penson, D. F., Cai, J., Groshen, S., Stein, J. P., Lieskovsky, G. and Skinner, D. G. (2006). Salvage radical prostatectomy: Quality-of-life outcomes and long-term oncological control of radiorecurrent prostate cancer. *J Urol, 176, 2025-31; discussion 2031-2.*

Tal, R., Alphs, H. H., Krebs, P., Nelson, C. J. and Mulhall, J. P. (2009). Erectile function recovery rate after radical prostatectomy: A meta-analysis. *J Sex Med, 6, 2538-46.*

Tal, R. and Mulhall, J. P. (2006). Sexual health issues in men with cancer. *Oncology (Williston Park), 20, 294-300; discussion 300, 303-4.*

Walsh, P. C. (2007). The discovery of the cavernous nerves and development of nerve-sparing radical retropubic prostatectomy. *J Urol, 177, 1632-5.*

References re: Prostate Cancer in HIV-Positive Patients in the Era of Highly-Active Antiretroviral Therapy (HAART)

American Cancer Society (2009). Cancer Facts and Figures. Atlanta, American Cancer Society.

"Joint United Nations Programme on HIV/AIDS (UNAIDS) and World Health Organization (WHO). AIDS Epidemic Update: (December 2007)."

Amir, H., E. E. Kaaya, et al. (2000). Breast cancer before and during the AIDS epidemic in women and men: A study of Tanzanian Cancer Registry data 1968 to 1996. *J Natl Med Assoc* 92(6): 301-5.

Andriole, G. L., E. D. Crawford, et al. (2009). Mortality results from a randomized prostate-cancer screening trial. *N Engl J Med* 360 (13): 1310-9.

Barrett-Connor, E. (1992). Lower endogenous androgen levels and dyslipidemia in men with non-insulin-dependent diabetes mellitus. *Ann Intern Med* 117(10): 807-11.

Bedimo, R. J., K. A. McGinnis, et al. (2009). Incidence of non-AIDS-defining malignancies in HIV-infected vs. non-infected patients in the HAART era: Impact of immunosuppression." *J Acquir Immune Defic Syndr.*

Biggar, R. J., K. A. Kirby, et al. (2004). Cancer risk in elderly persons with HIV/AIDS. *J Acquir Immune Defic Syndr* 36 (3): 861-8.

Bostwick, D. G., H. B. Burke, et al. (2004). Human prostate cancer risk factors. *Cancer* 101(10 Suppl): 2371-490.

Bratt, O., J. E. Damber, et al. (2002). Hereditary prostate cancer: Clinical characteristics and survival. *J Urol* 167(6): 2423-6.

Burgi, A., S. Brodine, et al. (2005). Incidence and risk factors for the occurrence of non-AIDS-defining cancers among human immunodeficiency virus-infected individuals. *Cancer* 104(7): 1505-11.

Calle, E. E., C. Rodriguez, et al. (2003). Overweight, obesity, and mortality from cancer in a prospectively studied cohort of U.S. adults. *N Engl J Med* 348(17): 1625-38.

Carter, H. B., P. C. Walsh, et al. (2002). Expectant management of nonpalpable prostate cancer with curative intent: preliminary results. *J Urol* 167(3): 1231-4.

Chiao, E. Y., S. E. Krown, et al. (2005). A population-based analysis of temporal trends in the incidence of squamous anal canal cancer in relation to the HIV epidemic. *J Acquir Immune Defic Syndr* 40(4): 451-5.

Christeff, N., S. Gharakhanian, et al. (1992). Evidence for changes in adrenal and testicular steroids during HIV infection. *J Acquir Immune Defic Syndr* 5(8): 841-6.

Clifford, G. M., J. Polesel, et al. (2005). Cancer risk in the Swiss HIV cohort study: Associations with immunodeficiency, smoking, and highly active antiretroviral therapy." *J Natl Cancer Inst* 97(6): 425-32.

Coussens, L. M. and Z. Werb (2002). Inflammation and cancer. *Nature 420*(6917): 860-7.

Crum, N. F., K. J. Furtek, et al. (2005). A review of hypogonadism and erectile dysfunction among HIV-infected men during the pre- and post-HAART eras: Diagnosis, pathogenesis, and management. *AIDS Patient Care STDS* 19(10): 655-71.

Crum, N. F., B. Hale, et al. (2002). Increased risk of prostate cancer in HIV infection? *AIDS* 16(12): 1703-4.

Crum, N. F., C. R. Spencer, et al. (2004). Prostate carcinoma among men with human immunodeficiency virus infection. *Cancer* 101(2): 294-9.

Crum-Cianflone, N., K. H. Hullsiek, et al. (2009). Trends in the incidence of cancers among HIV-infected persons and the impact of antiretroviral therapy: A 20-year cohort study. *AIDS* 23(1): 41-50.

Dal Maso, L., S. Franceschi, et al. (2003). Risk of cancer in persons with AIDS in Italy, 1985-1998. *Br J Cancer* 89(1): 94-100.

De Marzo, A. M., V. L. Marchi, et al. (1999). Proliferative inflammatory atrophy of the prostate: implications for prostatic carcinogenesis. *Am J Pathol* 155(6): 1985-92.

Demopoulos, B. P., E. Vamvakas, et al. (2003). Non-acquired immunodeficiency syndrome-defining malignancies in patients infected with human immunodeficiency virus. *Arch Pathol Lab Med* 127(5): 589-92.

Dobs, A. S. (1998). Androgen therapy in AIDS wasting.

Baillieres Clin Endocrinol Metab 12(3): 379-90.

Engels, E. A., R. M. Pfeiffer, et al. (2006). Trends in cancer risk among people with AIDS in the United States, 1980-2002. *AIDS* 20(12): 1645-54.

Epstein, J. I., D. W. Chan, et al. (1998). Nonpalpable stage T1c prostate cancer: Prediction of insignificant disease using free/total prostate specific antigen levels and needle biopsy findings. *J Urol* 160(6 Pt 2): 2407-11.

Feldman, J. G., S. J. Gange, et al. (2003). Serum albumin is a powerful predictor of survival among HIV-1-infected women. *J Acquir Immune Defic Syndr* 33(1): 66-73.

Freedland, S. J., M. K. Terris, et al. (2004). Obesity and biochemical outcome following radical prostatectomy for organ confined disease with negative surgical margins. *J Urol* 172(2): 520-4.

Frisch, M., R. J. Biggar, et al. (2001). Association of cancer with AIDS-related immunosuppression in adults. *JAMA* 285(13): 1736-45.

Gallagher, B., Z. Wang, et al. (2001). Cancer incidence in New York State acquired immunodeficiency syndrome patients. *Am J Epidemiol* 154(6): 544-56.

Gerard, L., L. Galicier, et al. (2003). Improved survival in HIV-related Hodgkin's lymphoma since the introduction of highly active antiretroviral therapy. *AIDS* 17(1): 81-7.

Gillanders, E. M., J. Xu, et al. (2004). Combined genome-wide scan for prostate cancer susceptibility genes. *J Natl Cancer Inst* 96(16): 1240-7.

Goedert, J. J., M. P. Purdue, et al. (2007). Risk of germ cell tumors among men with HIV/acquired immunodeficiency syndrome. *Cancer Epidemiol Biomarkers Prev* 16(6): 1266-9.

Goedert, J. J., C. Schairer, et al. (2006). Risk of breast, ovary, and uterine corpus cancers among 85,268 women with AIDS. *Br J Cancer* 95(5): 642-8.

Goldwasser, P. and J. Feldman (1997). Association of serum albumin and mortality risk. *J Clin Epidemiol* 50(6): 693-703.

Greene, K. L., P. C. Albertsen, et al. (2009). Prostate specific antigen best practice statement: 2009 update. *J Urol* 182(5): 2232-41.

Grubert, T. A., D. Reindell, et al. (2002). Rates of postoperative complications among human immunodeficiency virus-infected women who have undergone obstetric and gynecologic surgical procedures. *Clin Infect Dis* 34(6): 822-30.

Grulich, A. E., M. T. van Leeuwen, et al. (2007). Incidence of cancers in people with HIV/AIDS compared with immunosuppressed transplant recipients: A meta-analysis. *Lancet* 370(9581): 59-67.

Head, J. F., R. L. Elliott, et al. (1993). Evaluation of lymphocyte immunity in breast cancer patients. *Breast Cancer Res Treat* 26(1): 77-88.

Hengge, U. R. (2003). Testosterone replacement for hypogonadism: Clinical findings and best practices. *AIDS Read 13(12 Suppl)*: S15-21.

Hessol, N. A., S. Pipkin, et al. (2007). The impact of highly active antiretroviral therapy on non-AIDS-defining cancers among adults with AIDS. *Am J Epidemiol* 165(10): 1143-53.

Hessol, N. A., E. C. Seaberg, et al. (2004). Cancer risk among participants in the women's interagency HIV study. *J Acquir Immune Defic Syndr* 36(4): 978-85.

Hsiao, W., K. Anastasia, et al. (2009). Association between HIV status and positive prostate biopsy in a study of US veterans. *Scientific World Journal* 9: 102-8.

Huang, W. C., E. O. Kwon, et al. (2006). Radical prostatectomy in patients infected with human immunodeficiency virus. *BJU Int* 98(2): 303-7.

Jemal, A., R. Siegel, et al. (2009). Cancer statistics, 2009. *CA Cancer J Clin* 59(4): 225-49.

Klein, E. A. and R. Silverman (2008). Inflammation, infection, and prostate cancer. *Curr Opin Urol* 18(3): 315-9.

Kwan, D. J. and F. C. Lowe (1995). Genitourinary manifestations of the acquired immunodeficiency syndrome. *Urology* 45(1): 13-27.

Levinson, A., E. A. Nagler, et al. (2005). Approach to management of clinically localized prostate cancer in patients with human immunodeficiency virus. *Urology* 65(1): 91-4.

Loeb, S., K. A. Roehl, et al. (2006). Baseline prostate-specific antigen compared with median prostate-specific antigen for age group as predictor of prostate cancer risk in men younger than 60 years old. *Urology* 67(2): 316-20.

Lowe, F. C. (2008). Editorial Comment. *Urology* 72(5): 1138.

Ma, J., H. Li, et al. (2008). Prediagnostic body-mass index, plasma C-peptide concentration, and prostate cancer-specific mortality in men with prostate cancer: A long-term survival analysis. *Lancet Oncol* 9(11): 1039-47.

Mettlin, C., G. P. Murphy, et al. (1993). Characteristics of prostate cancers detected in a multimodality early detection program. The Investigators of the American Cancer Society-National Prostate Cancer Detection Project. *Cancer* 72(5): 1701-8.

Mylonakis, E., M. Paliou, et al. (2001). Plasma viral load testing in the management of HIV infection. *Am Fam Physician* 63(3): 483-90, 495-6.

Newcomer, L. M., J. L. Stanford, et al. (1997). Temporal trends in rates of prostate cancer: declining incidence of advanced stage disease, 1974 to 1994. *J Urol* 158(4): 1427-30.

Newnham, A., J. Harris, et al. (2005). The risk of cancer in HIV-infected people in southeast England: A cohort study. *Br J Cancer* 92(1): 194-200.

Ng, T., N. F. Stein, et al. (2008). Preliminary results of radiation therapy for prostate cancer in human immunodeficiency virus-positive patients. *Urology* 72(5): 1135-8; discussion 1138.

Pantanowitz, L., G. Bohac, et al. (2008). Human immunodeficiency virus-associated prostate cancer:

Clinicopathological findings and outcome in a multi-institutional study. *BJU Int* 101(12): 1519-23.

Patel, M. I., D. T. DeConcini, et al. (2004). An analysis of men with clinically localized prostate cancer who deferred definitive therapy. *J Urol* 171(4): 1520-4.

Patel, P., D. L. Hanson, et al. (2008). Incidence of types of cancer among HIV-infected persons compared with the general population in the United States, 1992-2003. *Ann Intern Med* 148(10): 728-36.

Phillips, A., A. G. Shaper, et al. (1989). Association between serum albumin and mortality from cardiovascular disease, cancer, and other causes. *Lancet* 2(8677): 1434-6.

Phillips, A. A. and J. E. Justman (2009). Screening HIV-infected patients for non-AIDS-defining malignancies. *Curr HIV/AIDS* Rep 6(2): 83-92.

Pitteloud, N., M. Hardin, et al. (2005). Increasing insulin resistance is associated with a decrease in Leydig cell testosterone secretion in men. *J Clin Endocrinol Metab* 90(5): 2636-41.

Quatan, N., S. Nair, et al. (2005). Should HIV patients be considered a high risk group for the development of prostate cancer? *Ann R Coll Surg Engl* 87(6): 437-8.

Raffi, F., J. M. Brisseau, et al. (1991). Endocrine function in 98 HIV-infected patients: A prospective study. *AIDS* 5(6): 729-33.

Richter, E., R. R. Connelly, et al. (2000). The role of pretreatment serum albumin to predict pathological stage and recurrence among radical prostatectomy cases. *Prostate*

Cancer Prostatic Dis 3(3): 186-190.

Rietschel, P., C. Corcoran, et al. (2000). Prevalence of hypogonadism among men with weight loss related to human immunodeficiency virus infection who were receiving highly active antiretroviral therapy. *Clin Infect Dis* 31(5): 1240-4.

Santillo, V. M. and F. C. Lowe (2005). Prostate cancer and the gay male. *Journal of Gay and Lesbian Psychotherapy* 9(1): 9-27.

Schackman, B. R., K. A. Gebo, et al. (2006). The lifetime cost of current human immunodeficiency virus care in the United States. *Med Care* 44(11): 990-7.

Schroder, F. H., J. Hugosson, et al. (2009). Screening and prostate-cancer mortality in a randomized European study. *N Engl J Med* 360(13): 1320-8.

Silva, M., P. R. Skolnik, et al. (1998). The effect of protease inhibitors on weight and body composition in HIV-infected patients. *AIDS* 12(13): 1645-51.

Silverberg, M. J., C. Chao, et al. (2009). HIV infection and the risk of cancers with and without a known infectious cause. *AIDS* 23(17): 2337-45.

Srirangam, A., R. Mitra, et al. (2006). Effects of HIV protease inhibitor ritonavir on Akt-regulated cell proliferation in breast cancer. *Clin Cancer Res* 12(6): 1883-96.

Stewart, T., S. C. Tsai, et al. (1995). Incidence of de-novo breast cancer in women chronically immunosuppressed after organ transplantation. *Lancet* 346(8978): 796-8.

Suzuki, M., A. Kanazawa, et al. (1999). A close association between insulin resistance and dehydroepiandrosterone sulfate in subjects with essential hypertension. *Endocr J* 46(4): 521-8.

Toniolo, A., C. Serra, et al. (1995). Productive HIV-1 infection of normal human mammary epithelial cells. *AIDS* 9(8): 859-66.

van Leeuwen, M. T., C. M. Vajdic, et al. (2009). Continuing declines in some but not all HIV-associated cancers in Australia after widespread use of antiretroviral therapy. *AIDS* 23(16): 2183-90.

Woolf, C. M. (1960). An investigation of the familial aspects of carcinoma of the prostate. *Cancer 13*: 739-44.

Wosnitzer, M. and F. Lowe (2010). Management of prostate cancer in HIV-positive patients. *Nature Reviews Urology* 7, (In press).

Wu, A. H., A. S. Whittemore, et al. (1995). Serum androgens and sex hormone-binding globulins in relation to lifestyle factors in older African-American, white, and Asian men in the United States and Canada. Cancer *Epidemiol Biomarkers Prev* 4(7): 735-41.

Wunder, D. M., N. A. Bersinger, et al. (2007). Hypogonadism in HIV-1-infected men is common and does not resolve during antiretroviral therapy. *Antivir Ther* 12(2): 261-5.

Zheng, S. L., J. Sun, et al. (2008). Cumulative association of five genetic variants with prostate cancer. *N Engl J Med* 358(9): 910-9.

References re: A Method for Identifying the Best Doctor and Treatment for Prostate Cancer

American Cancer Society (2010). www.csn.cancer.org/ forum, www.phoenix5.org/supportgroups.html.

Groopman, J. (2007), *How Doctors Think.* Houghton Mifflin Company, New York).

Howe, D. W. (1977), *Making the American Self: Jonathan Edwards to Abraham Lincoln.* Oxford University Press Publisher.

Kumar, S. M. (2009), *The Mindful Path Through Worry and Rumination: Letting go of Anxious and Depressive Thoughts.* New Harbinger Publications, Inc.

Le Doux, J. (1996), *The Emotional Brain: The Mysterious Underpinnings of Emotional Life.* Simon & Schuster Publishers

Levey, J. & Levey, M. (1999), *Simple Meditation and Relaxation.* Conari Press.

Malecare, (2010). www.Malecare.org

McNally, R. J. (2005), *Remembering Trauma.* Belknap Press.

Miller, W. R & C'deBaca, J. (2001), *Quantum Change: When Epiphanies and Sudden Insights Transform Ordinary Lives.* Guilford Press.

Perlman, G. (2005), Prostate cancer, the group, and me. In:

A Gay Men's Guide to Prostate Cancer. eds: G. Perlman & J. Drescher. Haworth Medical Press.

Papageorgiou, C. & Wells, A. (2005), Nature, functions, and beliefs about depressive rumination. In: *Depressive Rumination: Nature, Theory and Practice*. eds: C. Papageorgiou& A. Wells. John Wiley & Sons, Ontario, Canada.

Rock, D. (2009), *Your Brain at Work*. Harper Collins Publisher, New York.

Rogers, C. R. (1995), *On Becoming a Person: A Therapist's View of Psychotherapy*. Houghton Mifflin Publishers, New York.

Us TOO, (2010). http://www.ustoo.com.

References re: How a Gay Man Dealt with Personal Issues Before and After Radical Prostatectomy

Goldstone, S. (1999), *The Ins and Outs of Gay Sex, A Medical Handbook for Men*. New York: Dell Publishing.

Harris, J. (2005), Living with prostate cancer: One gay man's experience. *J. Gay & Lesbian Psychotherapy*, 9 (1/2): 109-117.

Marks, S. (1999), *Prostate & Cancer, A Family Guide to Diagnosis, Treatment & Survival*. Tucson: Fisher Book.

Martinez, R. (2005), Prostate cancer and sex. *J. Gay & Lesbian Psychotherapy*, 9 (1/2): 91-99

Masters, W. H. & Johnson, V. E. (1966), *Human Sexual Response*. Boston: Little, Brown and Co.

Miller, M. (2005) Identity and prostate cancer: Comments on a messy life. *J. Gay & Lesbian Psychotherapy*, 9 (1/2): 119-129.

Perlman, G. (2005), Glossary. *J. Gay & Lesbian Psychotherapy*, 9 (½): 1173-178.

Perlman, G. & Drescher, J. (Eds.) (2005), *A Gay Man's Guide to Prostate Cancer*. Binghamton, New York: The Haworth Medical Press.

Santillo, V. M. (2005), Prostate cancer diagnosis and treatment of a 33-year-old gay man. *J. Gay & Lesbian Psychotherapy*, 9 (1/2): 155-170.

Silverstein, C. & Picano, F. (2006), *The Joy of Gay Sex*. New York: Collins.

Zilbergeld, B. (1999), *The New Male Sexuality*. New York: Bantam Books.

References re: Robotic Radical Surgery

Carter, H. B. (2008). *The Johns Hopkins White Papers: Prostate Disorders*. Baltimore, MD: Johns Hopkins Medicine.

Jennings, Dana (2008). Real men get prostate cancer. New York: *The New York Times*, November 18.

Parkins, R.P. & Girven, H. Together with prostate cancer. *J. Gay & Lesbian Psychotherapy*, 9 (1/2): 137-146.

Tal, Ranaan (2012). Prostate cancer and sexual dysfunction in gay men. In: G. Perlman (ed.) *What Every Gay Man Needs to Know about Prostate Cancer*. New York: Magnus Books, Inc.

Walsh, P. (2001). *Dr. Patrick Walsh's Guide to Surviving Prostate Cancer*. New York: Warner Books.

Reference re: A Sex-Positive Gay Man Compares the Challenges of Being HIV-Positive, Having Prostate Cancer, and Life After it All

Jackson, L. (2005) Surviving yet another challenge. In: *A Gay Man's Guide to Prostate Cancer*, eds: G. Perlman & J. Drescher. New York, Haworth Medical Press, pp. 101-108.

Resources

In general, there is very little literature about how gay men's sexuality relates to prostate cancer or about gay men with prostate cancer in particular. Below are references that are specific to gay men; these are followed by more general books and essays about prostate cancer that may be helpful in understanding the disease. Next are recommended readings for health care providers. Finally, there is a list of websites for gay men, their caretakers, and health care providers.

Specific to Gay Men

Gerald Perlman, PhD & Jack Drescher, MD, (eds.), *A Gay Man's Guide to Prostate Cancer,* 2005, The Haworth Medical Press.

Blank, T.O. "Gay Men and Prostate Cancer: Invisible Diversity," *Journal of Clinical Oncology,* 2005, 3(12): 2593-2596.

General Resources for Men with Prostate Cancer

Mulhall, J.P. *Saving Your Sex Life: A Guide for Men with Prostate Cancer,* 2008, Hilton Publishing Company.

Scardino & Kelman, J. *Dr. Peter Scardino's Prostate Book: The Complete Guide to Overcoming Prostate Cancer,* Prostatitis, and BPH, 2006, Avery.

Walsh, P.C. & Farrar. J. *Dr. Patrick Walsh's Guide to Surviving Prostate Cancer*, Worthington, 2002, Grand Central Publishing.

Recommended Reading for Health Care Professionals

Blank T.O. "Gay Men and Prostate Cancer: Invisible Diversity. *Journal of Clinical Oncology*. 2005, 23(12): 2593-6. PMID: 15837977.

Magheli A, Burnett A. L. "Erectile Dysfunction Following Prostatectomy: Prevention and Treatment." *National Review of Urology*. 2009, 6(8): 415-27. PMID: 19657376.

Mulhall J.P. "Penile Rehabilitation Following Radical Prostatectomy." *Current Opinion in Urology*. 2008, 18(6): 613-20. PMID: 18832948.

Mulhall, J. P. *Sexual Function in the Prostate Cancer Patient*. Springer, 2009.

Shaiji T.A, Domes T, Brock G. "Penile Rehabilitation Following Treatment for Prostate Cancer: An Analysis of the Current State of the Art." *Canadian Urology Association Journal*. 2009, 3(1): 37-48. PMID: 19293974.

Tal R, Mulhall J.P. "Sexual Health Issues in Men with Cancer." *Oncology* (Williston Park). 2006, 20(3): 294-300; discussion 300, 303-4. PMID: 16629259.

Recommended Websites for Men with Prostate Cancer, Their Partners, Family and Friends

(A word of caution: Websites vary in quality, and often the

discussions can be overwhelming to the newly diagnosed patient. They can also be quite biased. Protect yourself by being aware of your information-overload limitations and the particular bias the website is presenting).

American Cancer Society: www.cancer.org

American Foundation of Urologic Diseases: www.afud.org

American Urological Association website: www.urologyhealth.org

Association of Peyronie's Disease Advocates website: www.peyroniesassoc.org

Cancer Care, Inc.: www.cancercare.org

Malecare: www.malecare.org. The website of a not-for-profit organization that has many essays of interest to gay men. This organization runs self-help groups for gay men with cancer around the world.

Menshealth: www.menshealth.about.com/od/gayhealth/ Gay-Concerns.htm. This is an information website for gay men seeking medical and psychological information pertinent to them.

Out with Cancer: www.outwithcancer.com. A website that is social, informative, and interactive; it is a subgroup of Malecare.

Mentors: www.yannow.org/Mentors/Russelw.htm. This is an interactional website based in Dallas, TX.

Prostate Cancer Advice: www.prostatecanceradvice.org. A website that allows you to ask questions about prostate cancer pertaining to gay men.

Prostate Cancer Foundation: www.pcf.org

Sexual Medicine Society of North America: www.sexhealthmatters.org

Us TOO: www.inspire.com/groups/ustoo-prostate-cancer/gay-men-with-prostate-cancer/ This is a website for gay men that is a subsection of Us TOO: a large self-help organization for men with prostate cancer.

Yahoo group: www.groups.yahoo.com/group/prostate.cancerandgaymen. An interactional website.

Recommended Websites for Health Care Professionals

International Society of Sexual Medicine: www.issm.info

Sexual Medicine Society of North America: www.smsna.org

American Urological Association: www.auanet.org

European Association of Urology: www.uroweb.org, www.uroweb.org

Acknowledgments

For helping bring this publication to fruition, I want to thank Bill Cohen, who steadfastly helped me find the right publisher for this book; Jack Drescher, MD, whose support and assistance goes way back; Darryl Mitteldorf, LCSW. In many ways he started the whole thing. Much appreciation goes to Don Weise from whom I have learned a great deal and who gently guided me through the process.

I want to express my gratitude to my friend and colleague Gil Tunnell, PhD. Not only did he contribute an essay about his own experience, he was instrumental in helping to edit several of the essays that appear in this volume. He asked that I let the reader know that it was his idea that I edit another book on prostate cancer and gay men. So thank you, Gil. A special thanks to David Trachtenberg, my life-partner, who provides me with a continuous source of love, support, and encouragement.

To all the authors who have contributed their time, effort, and patience, and whose enthusiasm for the project helped me through the rough spots, I am very grateful. Finally, to all the guys in Malecare's St. Vincent-Beth Israel's Gay Men's Prostate Cancer Group in New York City. You have been a joy to be with and an inspiration to me every time we met.

About the Editor

Gerald Perlman, PhD has been a Supervisor of Psychotherapy at the Albert Einstein College of Medicine, at Fordham, Pace, and Yeshiva Universities and at the City University of New York, as well as at the William Alanson White Institute where he received his certificate in Psychoanalysis. Dr. Perlman has written numerous essays and given many presentations on the practice of psychotherapy and the mental health issues of gay men. He is a Former Director of Psychology Internship Training at Manhattan Psychiatric Center in New York City. He is also former President of the New York Association of Gay and Lesbian Psychologists. Dr. Perlman was a member of the gay caucus of the New York State Psychological Association as well as at The William Alanson White Institute. Along with Jack Drescher, MD, he co-edited *A Gay Man's Guide to Prostate Cancer*. Dr. Perlman has also been on the editorial board of the *Journal of Gay & Lesbian Psychotherapy*. He was a Peer Reviewer for the Prostate Cancer Research Program under the auspices of the Department of Defense. Darryl Mitteldorf and Dr. Perlman have co-authored a manuscript concerning gay men with a variety of cancers that will appear in a volume entitled *Gay Lesbian Medical Association's Handbook on LGBT Health*, which covers many medical issues facing the LGBT community. In his private practice in New York, Dr. Perlman specializes in individual and couples therapy. For almost ten years (under the auspices of Malecare) he facilitated an ongoing, open-ended group for gay men who have been diagnosed with and/or treated for prostate cancer. The experiential essays written in this book come from some of the men who have been part of that group.

About the Professional Contributors

Marysol Asencio, DrPH received her doctorate from Columbia University's School of Public Health in 1994. She is an Associate Professor in the Department of Human Development and Family Studies concurrently with the Institute of Puerto Rican and Latino Studies at the University of Connecticut. She has written *Sex, Latina/o Sexuality: Probing Powers, Passions, Practices and Policies.*

Thomas O. Blank holds a PhD in Social Psychology from Columbia University and is a Professor at the University of Connecticut in the Department of Human Development and Family Studies. He is a Fellow of the Gerontological Society of America and the author or editor of five books and over forty essays. His primary interests concern the psychological and behavioral aspects of cancer survivorship, including gay men's attitudes and knowledge about prostate cancer.

Ashley Crawford earned her MA in Human Development and Family Studies in 2008 from the University of Connecticut. She is currently affiliated with the Department of Veterans Affairs in Newington, CT.

Lara Descartes was awarded her PhD in Anthropology from the University of Michigan in 2002. Formerly in the Department of Human Development and Family Studies at the University of Connecticut, she is now an Associate Professor of Family Studies at Brescia University College in London, Ontario. She co-authored *Media and Middle Class Moms and The Changing Landscape of Work and*

Family in the American Middle Class. Dr. Descartes is currently studying issues of family identity and parenting practices in single, lesbian mother families.

Steven Goldstone, MD is an Assistant Clinical Director of Surgery at Mt. Sinai School of Medicine in New York City.

Matthew Lemer, MD received his medical degree from Yale University and went on to do his residency in Urology at New York Presbyterian Hospital.

Franklin C. Lowe, MD, MPH is Professor of Clinical Urology at Columbia University, College of Physicians and Surgeons. He is also Associate Director at St. Luke's/Roosevelt Hospital in Manhattan. He has authored over 125 essays. His special interests include, prostate diseases, alternative medicine, HIV infection, and prostate cancer.

Darryl Mitteldorf, LCSW is an oncology social worker. He is the founder and executive director of Malecare, Inc., the first national gay men's cancer survivor support and advocacy nonprofit organization in the country. In addition to Malecare, he founded the LGBT Cancer Project: Out with Cancer. Widely published, and a speaker at numerous boards and conferences concerning cancer and gay men, he is also an advisor to several organizations. He received his BA from Swarthmore College and his MS and MSW from New York University.

Vincent M. Santillo, MD is currently in his residency in medicine at New York University/Bellevue Hospitals. The first part of his professional life was in finance, until a diagnosis of prostate cancer at age thirty-three spurred him to pursue a career in medicine. He received his BS in Economics from the University of Pennsylvania, an MBA from Columbia University, and his MD from Columbia University, College of Physicians and Surgeons, where he was inducted into the Gold Humanism Honor Society.

Raanan Tal, MD is a senior urologic surgeon at the Male Sexual Medicine and Reproductive Program at Rabin Medical Center in Israel. He was trained at Memorial Sloan-Kettering Cancer Center in New York City with a focus on the medical and surgical treatment of sexual dysfunctions in men coping with cancer. Dr. Tal is a member of the American Urological Association and the International Society for Sexual Medicine. He is in private practice in Tel-Aviv, Israel.

Matthew Wosnitzer, MD is chief resident in urology at Columbia University Medical Center, where he has studied HIV-associated nephropathy.

About the Experiential Contributors

Joe Davenport is a retired Purchasing Director for New York City Transit. He received a BA and an MBA from Pace University. He has been in a twenty-year relationship with his partner, Don.

John Dalzell, MS is a former news reporter and currently writes about the behavioral sciences. He also works as an organizational psychologist and educator in New York City.

"Charles Godfry" is a pseudonym for a sixty-year-old gay man who is a senior vice president at a major real estate firm in New York. He received his BA in Architectural History at a large university in the Midwest, and came to New York City in the late '70s to participate in the Historic Preservation Program at Columbia University

Lidell Jackson is a retired ballet and Broadway dancer. He is the co-founder and organizer of Jacks of Color, a safe-sex club for men of color and their friends. He has been a longstanding political activist in the New York City LGBTQI community. Born and raised in Memphis, Tennessee, he holds a BA in Applied Mathematics from Brown University.

Frank John is a fifty-seven-year-old, spiritual gay man who was educated in the Catholic school system; Frank went on to a career in corporate human resources. He left that to become a licensed massage therapist.

"Paul Jarod" is a pseudonym for a man who works as a marketing consultant in New York City. He received his

MA from Fairleigh Dickinson University. In his spare time he likes to hike and to create personal travelogues from his visits around the globe.

"James Larsen" is a pseudonym for a self-described farm boy from Colorado who made his way to New York City over twenty years ago. He studied comparative literature at Loyola University in Chicago, and currently works as a legal assistant and freelance artist.

Roberto Martinez is a doctoral candidate at CUNY Graduate Center. A former board member of Latino Gay Men of New York, he is currently Assistant Director for Graduate Advising and Student Services in the Department of Teaching and Learning at New York University Steinhardt School of Education.

"Mark Red" is a pseudonym for a man who has worked in the advertising industry for more than thirty years. Because he has not told his elderly parents about his health issues nor that he is in a 12-step program, and recognizing the complications it might create for possible employees he has chosen to remain anonymous.

Milton Sonday, who proudly resides in Brooklyn, NY and Berks County, PA, received his MFA from Carnegie Mellon University. He is a former curator of textiles at the Cooper-Hewitt Museum and is currently a freelance artist and textile historian.

Gil Tunnell, PhD is an Adjunct Associate Professor of Psychology and Education at Teacher's College of Columbia University. He is also a senior faculty member at the Accelerated Experiential Dynamic Psychotherapy Institute in New York City. Dr. Tunnell co-authored *Couples Therapy with Gay Men*. He is a Former Director of

Family Therapy Training at Beth Israel Medical Center in New York City as well as a former Senior Psychologist and Clinical Assistant Professor of Psychiatry at New York University. Gil was also Chair of the Task Force on AIDS of the New York State Psychological Association.

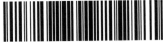

Made in the USA
Charleston, SC
14 March 2013